Positive Options for Living with Your Ostomy

About the Author

Dr. Craig A. White is a Clinical Psychologist and Research Fellow at the Department of Psychological Medicine, University of Glasgow, Scotland. Dr. White graduated with a first-class honours degree in psychology from the University of Glasgow in 1992 and then completed his doctorate in clinical psychology at the University of Manchester, England, in 1995.

His clinical and research interests are in psychological adjustment to physical illness, particularly cancer and adjustment to changed appearance. He is the author of a major textbook on the treatment of psychological aspects of medical problems and has published his work on adjustment to ostomy surgery in surgical, nursing, and psychological journals. He is involved with teaching and research on psychosocial adjustment to ostomy surgery and regarded as an expert on the psychology of ostomy care.

FOR ADAM

Ordering

Trade bookstores in the U.S. and Canada please contact:

Publishers Group West
1700 Fourth Street, Berkeley CA 94710
Phone: (800) 788-3123   Fax: (510) 528-3444

Hunter House books are available at bulk discounts for textbook course adoptions;
to qualifying community, healthcare, and government organizations; and for special
promotions and fund-raising. For details please contact:

Special Sales Department
Hunter House Inc., PO Box 2914, Alameda CA 94501-0914
Phone: (510) 865-5282   Fax: (510) 865-4295
E-mail: ordering@hunterhouse.com

Individuals can order our books from most bookstores, by calling
(800) 266-5592, or from our website at **www.hunterhouse.com**

Positive Options
for Living
with Your
Ostomy

Self-Help and Treatment

Dr. Craig A. White

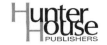

Hunter House
PUBLISHERS

Hunter House Inc., Publishers
PO Box 2914
Alameda CA 94501-0914

First published in Great Britain in 1997 by
Sheldon Press, SPCK, Marylebone Road, London NW1 4DU

Library of Congress Cataloging-in-Publication Data

White, Craig A.
Positive options for living with your ostomy : self-help and treatment / Craig A. White
    p. cm.   Includes index.
ISBN 0-89793-358-3 (paper) — ISBN 0-89793-359-1 (cloth)
1. Ostomates—Popular works. 2. Enterostomy—Popular works. 3. Nephrostomy—Popular works. I. Title.
RD540 .W525 2001
617.5'5—dc21   2001043083

Project Credits

Cover Design: Brian Dittmar Graphic Design
Book Production: Hunter House
Copy Editor: Kelley Blewster
Proofreader: John David Marion
Indexer: Kathy Talley-Jones
Acquisitions Editor: Jeanne Brondino
Associate Editor: Alexandra Mummery
Sales and Marketing Assistant: Earlita K. Chenault
Publicity Manager: Sara Long
Customer Service Manager: Christina Sverdrup
Warehousing & Shipping: Lakdhon Lama
Administrator: Theresa Nelson
Computer Support: Peter Eichelberger
Publisher: Kiran S. Rana

Printed and Bound by Bang Printing, Brainerd, Minnesota

Manufactured in the United States of America
9 8 7 6 5 4 3 2 1   First Edition   02 03 04 05 06

Contents

Important Note

The material in this book is intended to provide a review of resources and information related to living with an ostomy. Every effort has been made to provide accurate and dependable information. However, professionals in the field may have differing opinions, and change is always taking place. Any of the treatments described herein should be undertaken only under the guidance of a licensed health-care practitioner. The author, editors, and publishers cannot be held responsible for any error, omission, professional disagreement, outdated material, or adverse outcomes that derive from use of any of the treatments or information resources in this book, either in a program of self-care or under the care of a licensed practitioner.

Foreword

Even when it enhances a patient's life, having an ostomy is a major, life-altering event in both physical and psychological aspects. Decisions on the need for an ostomy are often made as part of life-saving treatment. During these stressful times, there may not be enough time or interest to explore all the ramifications associated with ostomies. Even when information is provided, patients may not be ready to absorb all the material presented. This may be due to some component of denial or desire to delay some of these issues until the patient begins to recover from his or her illness. Finally, the magnitude of alterations may not be fully appreciated until one actually lives with an ostomy. These problems have a greater impact if the patient has unresolved emotional or psychological issues prior to receiving an ostomy.

Colorectal surgeons are dedicated to improving patients' lives. We continuously work toward eliminating the need for permanent as well as temporary ostomies. When ostomies are required, we lead a team of providers whose goal is to produce the best possible stoma which has the least impact on the patient's lifestyle. Enterostomal therapy nurses are major participants in this team effort. They provide invaluable support to ostomates and their families and often have more time to spend with patients. Another valuable resource and advocate for ostomates in the United States is the United Ostomy Associaton. This volunteer group of patients with ostomies and their families provide information, visitations, and serve as a rallying point for ostomy concerns.

Dr. White has extensive experience in helping patients adjust to life changes. As a psychologist, he brings a unique perspective to patients' concerns. His informative book provides valuable information on an aspect of medical care that has been underserved by published material for patients as well as professionals. The book is easy and enjoyable to read and well-organized. After providing the reader with basic information on the intestinal system and basic medical care, specific details of ostomies and ostomy care are presented. Perhaps most importantly, there are extensive discussions on the emotional aspects of coping with ostomies and social situations. The book also provides the reader with information on many additional sources of information and help. I learned a lot from this book and I would highly recommend it to my patients and other health care providers.

DAVID E. BECK, M.D.
Chairman, Department of Colon and Rectal Surgery
Ochsner Clinic, New Orleans
and
Chairman, Medical Advisory Committtee
United Ostomy Association

Preface

As a colorectal surgeon, I see patients with various types of ostomies on a daily basis. It is interesting to me how fearful patients are about ostomies before surgery and how well managed and comfortable they can become with them after surgery. Although no patient would choose to have an ostomy if they had an alternative, when patients are instructed properly in the management of an ostomy and have their questions answered in a timely and appropriate fashion, adjustment is easy and quality of life is very high.

Dr. White has made a real contribution by tapping a body of information that has not heretofore been readily available. Patients communicate with each other and develop information that has not been taught to the physician. Dr. White has assembled much of this information into this book which should give patients a running start on adjusting to their ostomy. Continued interaction with other patients who have an ostomy and who have learned the techniques of management and adjustment through the college of "hard knocks" will be the source of ongoing education for patients as they work with their ostomy. Overall, the ostomy is not something to be feared, but rather another alternative that can be perceived as "normal" and which allows the patient to live a long and normal life.

Readers will find this book easy to read, pragmatic in its approach, and will refer to it frequently during the early months of their ostomy. It is a great resource to help patients through what is initially perceived to be a difficult time but can ultimately result in a very high quality of life for many years.

ROBERT W. BEART, JR., M.D.

Acknowledgments

My work in this area was inspired by Lynne Park.

The UK edition of this book was dedicated to my wife Gwen in acknowledgement of her unfailing support for my work and to my parents for their support and encouragement. I also thanked Ann and Andrew McPhail. I am no less grateful to all of them for the part they continue to play in my life, but I have dedicated the American edition of this book to another light in my life—my son, Adam.

I am grateful to Agnes Walls, clinical nurse specialist in stoma care; Jane Collier, dietician; John McGregor, consultant surgeon; and James Russell, consultant radiologist (retired), who have all provided advice and information incorporated within parts of this book. I wish to acknowledge the assistance of the staff of Hunter House Publications for their work in preparing this U.S. edition. Special thanks to Wendel Brown for research conducted in connection with this publication.

Introduction

Between 42,000 and 65,000 ostomy surgeries are performed each year in the United States. An estimated 750,000 Americans wear an ostomy-care applicance. *Positive Options for Living with Your Ostomy* is concerned with the practical and emotional aspects of living with particular types of ostomies called colostomies, ileostomies, and urostomies. It does not cover the issues relating to other types of ostomies, such as gastrostomies or tracheostomies, and it does not provide information on ostomy care for children.

An ostomy is an opening created by a surgeon on the abdomen to allow waste material (urine or feces) to be expelled. An ostomy is usually necessary when the normal bodily systems for expelling waste material are not functioning, due to an accident or a disease. (The differences between colostomies, ileostomies, and urostomies are explained later in the book.) You may already have an ostomy and will therefore know that this involves a major change in the way your body works. If you do not have an ostomy, or are about to have one formed, I'm sure you can imagine that changing the way your body gets rid of waste material is a major issue. This book is about the physiological and psychological changes involved following ostomy surgery, how to cope with these changes, and how to get back to a normal life.

Many informational pamphlets about adjustment to ostomy surgery are extremely positive. Some show pictures of ostomy patients (otherwise known as *ostomates*) playing tennis or sitting with their family around them smiling. I am not suggesting that these pictures misrepresent what can be achieved by most ostomy patients after their surgery. However, I believe that health-care professionals should provide more explicit acknowledgement that life with an ostomy can be challenging at first, that you are not unusual if you have problems or worries, and that any problems which crop up can usually be dealt with in a straightforward way. I hope that by reading this book you will learn about some of the possible problems and that you can either prevent them from happening in the first place, or identify them early and develop coping strategies or ways of resolving them.

Ostomy operations are usually lifesaving procedures. They are almost always performed because there is no alternative. Medical staff recommend an ostomy operation if a disease or physical problem is going to worsen without the surgery. The fact that ostomy operations are lifesaving *can* make it easier for some people to accept an ostomy. However, I know some people who have had an ostomy operation and, despite the knowledge that they would be dead without the ostomy, still find it difficult to live with. In other words, just because it saved your life does not mean that you have to like it. Life with an ostomy can be difficult. This book will help you lessen the problems of life with an ostomy and appreciate and enjoy the new life provided by the ostomy operation.

Approximately ten years ago, I realized that very little had been written by psychologists on adjustment to ostomy surgery—and thus I decided to begin some psychologically based research in this area. This is how my interest in adjustment to ostomy surgery developed, and it was the source of the initial idea for this book. In writing the book, I have tried to combine the "common wisdom" from within the field of ostomy care with aspects of my work as a clinical psychologist—to provide practical information on ostomy care as well as some unique ideas of my own about dealing with life with an ostomy. Research into the psychology of living with an ostomy shows that most people who have had the operation experience a considerable amount of worry and concern as they adjust to life with an ostomy. For most people, this is part of a normal adjustment process following a major illness, major surgery, and the experience of a change in the way their body looks and works. But other people who have undergone ostomy surgery—approximately 25 percent of those who have had an ostomy operation—

experience more serious psychological symptoms after the surgery. People who have experienced psychological problems before ostomy surgery are more likely to experience psychological problems after ostomy surgery. If this applies to you, then you should inform your doctor or nurse so that extra support can be provided. This book has been written for both groups of people: those who have minor difficulties which are part of normal adjustment and those who have more severe and incapacitating problems.

Positive Options for Living with Your Ostomy is primarily for the person who has had an ostomy operation—though it is also for anyone who wants to learn more about what an ostomy is and how it can affect quality of life. It will be useful if you or someone you know is to have an ostomy operation, or if you are involved in the care of someone with an ostomy. It aims to provide information on the practical and emotional aspects of coping with life after ostomy surgery. It is not meant to be a substitute for the skilled advice and postoperative care provided by doctors, ostomy-care nurses, surgeons, and other health-care professionals. I hope that it will reinforce and complement the advice and help given by those professionals. Not all health-care professionals are knowledgeable about ostomy care, as they may only occasionally come into contact with an ostomy patient. Most general practioners will have only a couple of ostomy patients within their practice and may not be able to advise you on all aspects of ostomy care.

As a clinical psychologist, I am especially interested in promoting the best possible degree of psychological adjustment following ostomy operations. This book has therefore been written with psychological adjustment in mind—to provide the kind of information and advice that doctors, surgeons, and nurses may not give, and to do so in a way that can be of practical use to someone who is getting used to life with an ostomy.

Research has suggested that satisfaction with information is vital in helping people come to terms with surgery. I hope this book will include all the information you could possibly need to get used to life with an ostomy. In addition to providing general information on life after ostomy surgery, I have tried to highlight problems which may need more than advice from a book. Certain physical or psychological problems require expert professional help. Unfortunately, a large proportion of ostomy patients with psychological problems do not receive professional help, as their nurses and doctors fail to notice such problems in their patients. I hope this book might be of some help if you have been suffering in silence and that you might receive the right kinds of support and help as a result of what you read here. If you have any doubt at all about whether to speak to a nurse or doctor about a problem, err on the side of caution: Do not hesitate to contact a professional for advice.

What Is in This Book?

Like other surgical procedures, an ostomy operation has wide-ranging effects on many different aspects of a person's life and is carried out to cure or help alleviate the symptoms of particular diseases. You need to know about the disease and its symptoms and why an ostomy operation is being suggested in preference to another type of operation. Unlike many other operations, having an ostomy involves having an ostomy-care appliance ("bag" or "pouch") and learning how to manage an ostomy-care routine. So, certain aspects of getting used to life with an ostomy are common to recovering from any form of surgery—but there are many aspects unique to this type of operation.

Chapter 1 gives an overview of the anatomy and function of the human digestive and urinary systems; it is usually diseases in these bodily systems that are treated by an ostomy operation. You need to understand how these body systems work if you are to understand why an ostomy is a helpful treatment and how the surgeon creates an ostomy. Chapter 2 outlines details of the different types of ostomies covered in this book and how ostomies are created. Chapter 3 provides detailed explanations of the various medical tests that might be carried out before and after the ostomy operation, along with suggestions on getting the information you want about your disease, symptoms, and treatment. Descriptions of medical personnel you may encounter while in the hospital are also given in this chapter.

Life with an ostomy means life with an ostomy-care appliance. Chapter 4 includes all you need to know about ostomy-care appliances and how to get used to them without major problems. This chapter also includes some helpful charts for you to complete to monitor your confidence in changing the appliance and to keep notes on your experiences with different appliances. There is also a troubleshooting guide for appliance problems.

Thoughts about the ostomy can contribute to problematic feelings, and Chapter 5 looks at how these feelings and thoughts can become negatively biased. This chapter includes some questions to help you develop a thinking style that is less negatively biased about the ostomy. The common emotional reactions to ostomy surgery are explained in Chapter 6, along with some simple techniques to deal with them. The main focus of this chapter is on identifying the problematic thoughts underlying anxiety and depression, including details on how to change these problem thoughts to help you feel better.

The next two chapters focus on the effect ostomy operations can have on relationships. Chapter 7 deals with the effects of ostomy surgery on relationships with other people in general, and on social interactions. The impact of ostomy surgery on intimate relationships and sexual functioning is covered in Chapter 8, along with details on the human sexual response and common sexual problems. Chapter 9 covers some important aspects of enjoying life with an ostomy; various issues relating to travel, diet, work, sleep, and sports are addressed for those who desire advice on these aspects of adjustment. You will find useful resources and information on further reading at the end of the book.

Since I have become interested in the psychological aspects of ostomy care, I have received some letters from patients who have developed problems in adjusting to life with an ostomy. I don't wish to discourage anyone from writing to me about how they have coped, the problems they have had (or are having), or how they have found this book useful. However, there are limits to the help that can be offered at a distance. If you are looking for individual help, my advice is always to discuss your concerns with your family doctor first of all. You may wish to show your nurse or doctor some of the information and coping strategies outlined in the book. He or she might then be able to help you apply them to your own problems and work through them. He or she will also be able to put you in touch with a specialist in ostomy care or a specialist in psychological problems.

Summary

Having an ostomy operation involves a major change in the way the human body deals with waste materials.

This book includes all you need to know about getting used to life with an ostomy.

Most people who have undergone an ostomy operation have some worries or concerns after surgery. These range from reactions that are part of the normal adjustment process to those which are part of more serious psychological problems requiring treatment.

This book is not meant to be a substitute for the professional advice given to ostomy patients by doctors, nurses, and other health professionals. It aims to provide you with accurate information and to help you prevent, identify, and cope with ostomy-related concerns as well as you possibly can.

Chapter 1

The Digestive and Urinary Systems

Ostomies are not often talked about. Because of this, many people go through life without ever having heard a straightforward, realistic discussion about them. Sometimes we get ideas based on what we have heard from other people or what we have read in magazines.

To understand what happens when an ostomy is formed, we need first to have some idea about how the digestive system and/or the urinary system works. This is because an ostomy operation is usually the result of a problem with the digestive or urinary system. This chapter describes how both of these important bodily systems work and then outlines some information on the common diseases that can affect each system.

The Digestive System

The way in which we digest food seems so automatic—we don't need to think about it after we have swallowed. However, a lot happens in our bodies after we have swallowed our food. The main job of the digestive system is to break down (digest) food into simpler parts so that the important nutrients our bodies need can be taken into (absorbed into) the bloodstream. These nutrients are

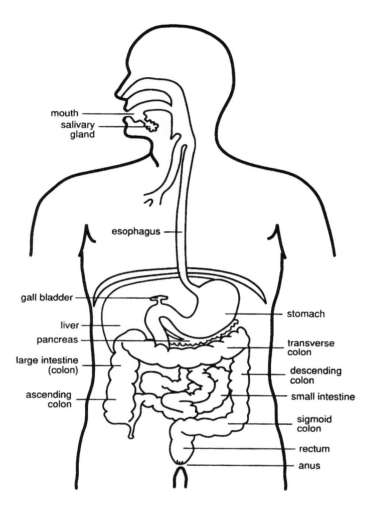

mouth
salivary
gland

esophagus

gall bladder

liver
pancreas

large intestine
(colon)

ascending
colon

stomach

transverse
colon

descending
colon

small intestine

sigmoid
colon

rectum

anus

Figure 1. The Digestive System

absorbed as the food makes its way through our digestive system. After the nutrients have been absorbed into the blood, they can then be carried throughout the body via the bloodstream to the parts that need them most. Each part of the body takes what it needs for its own growth and repair. The digestive system also provides us with a way of getting rid of the waste products that remain after our bodies have used all the nutrients they need. The main parts of the digestive system are outlined in Figure 1.

After we have put food into our mouths, it needs to be broken down before it can pass to the next stage in the digestive process. We begin to break the food down by chewing it. Saliva, produced by the salivary glands, mixes with the chewed-up food to break down the food even more. Once the food has been chewed and mixed with the saliva, it is then ready to pass down the esophagus. The esophagus is a flattened muscular tube about 30–40 centimeters (12–16 inches) in length. The food travels down the esophagus into the stomach. When the food reaches the stomach, the next stage of the digestive process—called gastric digestion—can begin.

The stomach is a like a hollow bag in which food is mixed with digestive juices and churned up (a bit like a blender). The stomach does this mixing by making slow churning movements. The juices from the stomach (called gastric juices) and the food are thoroughly mixed together until the mixture has a gruel-like consistency. This gruel-like fluid is called chyme. It can take anywhere between one and six hours for the food you put into your mouth to be changed into chyme, depending on what you have eaten. A simple meal, such as a cup of tea with bread and butter, is digested in the stomach in about one hour, whereas a meal that contains eggs, milk, or meat might take three hours. A heavy dinner, which might include several courses, can take up to seven hours to digest fully in the stomach and become chyme.

The chyme then passes from the stomach into the small intestine, where digestion continues. The small intestine is a long, twisting maze of tube about 6 yards in length. The chyme is converted by fluids from other parts of the body into a yellow, creamy fluid called chyle. The chyle moves along the small intestine, and as it moves, all the nutrients from the food are absorbed through the walls of the intestine. Most of the goodness from food materials is absorbed in the small intestine. The leftovers now have to be dealt with by the other parts of the digestive system.

The remains of the food keep passing along the digestive system, moving from the small intestine to the large intestine. The large intestine is another long tube, about 1.5 yards long, and wider than the small intestine. This is where the final stages of digestion occur. The main job of the large intestine (or colon) is to absorb water and other important chemicals into our bodies from the food. When the colon has done this, waste material (called feces) is all that remains. The feces are moved down the colon by sweeping muscular contractions called peristalsis. You may have noticed that the urge to pass feces comes on after eating food. This is because eating can trigger these muscular contractions. The contractions cause waste to move further down the digestive system. The feces pass down to the rectum, which acts like a storage tank for the waste material—and for any food that could not be digested as it travelled through the digestive system. Once the rectum is full, we get the desire to pass the waste material. When it is convenient, we get rid of the waste by the relaxation of the internal and external muscles of the rectum. The abdominal and pelvic-floor muscles are contracted, and the waste material is then expelled through the anus—the opening at the end of the rectum. This is the final stage of the digestive process.

The Urinary System

The main parts of the urinary system are shown in Figure 2. The kidneys are complex organs that filter out waste products from the blood. After they have done this, they flush out waste material through two narrow tubes called ureters. The ureters feed into the bladder, a hollow organ in the lower part of the abdomen that acts as a storage area for urine. Urine is the liquid waste that is made by the kidneys when they have cleaned the blood supply. When the bladder is almost full of urine, a message is sent to the brain telling it that the bladder is nearly full. When it is appropriate to do so, relaxing the sphincter muscle causes urine to flow out of the urethra—an action similar to when we relax the muscles above the anus to let the feces out.

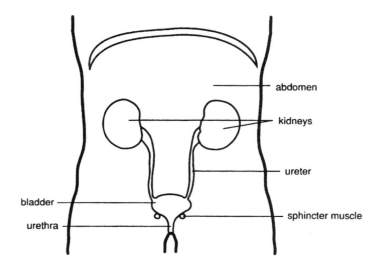

Figure 2. The Urinary System

Problems with the Digestive and Urinary Systems

Now that we have seen how these systems work, we will look at some of the main diseases that can cause problems with them. Sometimes these diseases are treated by an operation in which an ostomy is formed. Understanding the main diseases will make it easier to understand why an ostomy operation might be performed to help with a particular disease.

The following digestive-system diseases are the ones most commonly treated by an ostomy operation. Some of the symptoms mentioned can be caused by other, less serious, conditions.

Ulcerative Colitis

Ulcerative colitis is a disease in which the lining of the large intestine (including the rectum) becomes inflamed and ulcerated. These ulcers can weep and bleed. Ulcerative colitis can occur at any age, though people between ages twenty and forty are most commonly affected. Its main symptoms are diarrhea mixed with blood, mucus and/or pus, stomachache, loss of appetite, sickness, weight loss, a frequent need to empty the bowels, and pain at the anus. This disease tends to come and go. Sufferers have periods between flare-ups when they feel completely well—these are called periods of remission. The treatment for most patients with ulcerative colitis is drugs. Sometimes an operation is needed because the drugs are not working or because the ulcerative colitis has worsened very quickly. People with ulcerative colitis have a higher chance of getting bowel or rectal cancer—they may have an ostomy operation because of this higher risk.

Crohn's Disease

Crohn's disease is also an inflammatory bowel disease. Like ulcerative colitis, it can occur at any age. Unlike ulcerative colitis, Crohn's disease can occur anywhere in the digestive system, from mouth to anus. In this disease, part of the digestive system becomes inflamed and develops ulcers. The most commonly affected area of the digestive system is the last part of the small intestine (terminal ileum) and part of the colon or rectum. The symptoms of Crohn's disease are bleeding from the anus, colicky abdominal pain after meals, weight loss, diarrhea with mucus and/or pus, fever, nausea, vomiting, lethargy, and loss of appetite. Many people who have Crohn's disease need to have an operation. If the disease affects the small bowel, this operation will usually involve removal of diseased bowel. An ostomy operation is much more likely in a case of Crohn's disease that affects the large bowel.

Familial Polyposis Coli (Gardner's Syndrome)

Familial polyposis coli is a condition in which the large intestine develops polyps (pronounced "pollups") that are at risk of becoming cancerous. This disease is inherited. Every child of a parent with this disease stands a fifty-fifty chance of developing it himself.

Children of parents who have this condition need to have regular checkups when they reach their teenage years to see if they have developed any polyps.

Diverticular Disease

Diverticular disease is common after the age of forty. It affects about one-third of people over the age of sixty. Someone with diverticular disease may have few symptoms; consequently, they may not know they have it. A lack of fiber in the diet can be a contributory factor to the development of this disease. The lack of fiber results in small, hard bowel movements that are difficult to move along the bowel. This produces high pressure in the bowel, which causes pouches to form. These pouches, called diverticulae, develop outward through the bowel wall. Feces can become trapped in these pouches and can cause irritation. If this happens, inflammation, pain, altered bowel habits, abdominal distension, and bleeding can result. A high-fiber diet may be recommended, or sometimes an operation is suggested. This does not necessarily involve an ostomy, although this is more likely if the surgery is for an emergency, as in the case of diverticular perforation.

Colorectal Cancer

Colorectal cancer (sometimes called bowel cancer or rectal cancer) is a disease wherein cancer (malignant) cells are found in the large intestine and/or rectum. In the United States, it is the fourth most commonly diagnosed cancer and ranks second among cancer deaths. It usually comes on gradually, and symptoms may not occur until the later stages of the disease. The symptoms of colorectal cancer are the passing of mucus or slime from the anus, distension of the abdomen, abdominal pain, a change in bowel habits, bleeding from the anus, or a sense of fullness in the back passage. The main treatment for bowel and rectal cancer is the removal of the part which is affected; this may or may not mean that an ostomy operation is needed.

Cancer of the Anus

Cancer of the anus is an uncommon cancer. Symptoms of this cancer can include bleeding from the rectum, pain in the area around the anus, a lump near the anus, and itchiness or a discharge of fluid from the anus.

Cancer of the Bladder

Cancer of the bladder is a disease wherein cancer (malignant) cells are found in the bladder. Blood in the urine (called hematuria), frequent urination, a burning sensation when passing urine, and a feeling of needing to urinate although nothing comes out are all common symptoms of bladder cancer. Bladder cancer has the highest incidence rates in industrialized countries such as the United States and Canada; its incidence is lower in the UK.

Other Problems

Besides being brought on by disease, problems with the digestive or urinary systems can also result from accidents in which damage or injury has occurred to the anal sphincter or large bowel, or following pelvic fractures involving damage to the rectum that disrupts the proper functioning of the digestive or urinary system. Additionally, radiotherapy treatment for cancers can cause damage to important digestive or urinary organs, and this damage in turn can cause problems. Finally, problems with the urinary system can also be caused by diseases of the nervous system, such as multiple sclerosis.

Summary

This chapter has covered important information about how our digestive and urinary systems work. It has also provided some details of the diseases that can cause problems with these important systems. Sometimes these diseases are treated by arranging for the person to have an operation in which an ostomy is formed.

The digestive system is responsible for taking in the food we eat, making sure our bodies get all the important nutrients they need, and then getting rid of the waste material.

The main parts of the digestive system are the esophagus, stomach, small intestine, large intestine, rectum, and anus.

The urinary system deals with the liquid waste from our bodies after our kidneys have filtered out waste materials from our blood supply.

The main parts of the urinary system are the kidneys, ureters, bladder, and urethra.

The main diseases that affect the digestive system and which may need an ostomy operation include ulcerative colitis, Crohn's disease, polyps, diverticular disease, and colorectal cancer.

The main disease that affects the urinary system and which may need an ostomy operation is cancer of the bladder.

The next chapter will explain the different types of ostomies and how they are created.

Chapter 2

Ostomies: The Basics

This chapter describes the most common types of ostomies and outlines what happens when a surgeon performs an ostomy operation. It is crucial that you understand why an ostomy operation is recommended, and that you are able to talk to your doctors and nurses without becoming confused. The main ostomies covered in this chapter are a colostomy, an ileostomy, and a urostomy.

The terms *ostomy* and *stoma* have different meanings. An ostomy refers to the surgically created opening in the body for the discharge of bodily waste. A stoma is the actual part of the body which can be seen protruding through the abdominal wall. The terms used for ostomy operations can be broken down to help us understand them. The second part of each word, *-stomy*, means "to form a new opening or outlet." The word *colostomy* is made up of *colon* and *-ostomy*. The colon is the large intestine; the whole word thus means "to form a new outlet for the large intestine." The word *ileostomy* is made up of *ileum*—which is a part of the small intestine—and *-stomy*, and thus describes the formation of a new opening for the small intestine. The word *urostomy* is made up of *ur-* and *-stomy* and refers to the creation of a new outlet for urine.

One common factor in all ostomy operations is that a new opening or outlet is created by the surgeon. The other common factor is that a part of the inside of the body is brought to the surface to make the new opening. This is called a stoma. Stomas are moist and red in color (like the inside of your mouth). They have no nerve endings and are not sensitive to being touched. Stomas may sometimes make a sort of gurgling noise when they are producing waste material or when gas escapes.

What Is a Colostomy?

Colostomy is the name given to the opening made during an operation when the large intestine (colon) is brought to the surface of the abdomen so that waste material comes out there instead of travelling down to the rectum (as described in Chapter 1). A colostomy is the most common type of ostomy. It is usually formed after treatment for colorectal cancer or cancer of the anus. To make a colostomy, the surgeon cuts a hole in the patient's lower abdomen and sews a piece of bowel to the skin surface. This piece of bowel forms the stoma. Instead of the large intestine travelling all the way down to the rectum, it has been diverted to the surface of the body. If the rectum is not removed, then the surgeon may also bring the cut end of the rectum to the surface of the body. This small opening is called a mucus fistula; it discharges only mucus. The colostomy is usually situated to the left of and just below the navel.

Another circumstance under which a colostomy operation might be carried out is when there has been an injury to the rectum that cannot be repaired. When the rectum has been damaged during an illness, the surgeon sometimes removes the anus and the lower part of the rectum. When the rectum, anus, and part of the colon are removed in this way and a colostomy is formed, the operation is called an abdominoperineal resection.

After an operation of this type, people may experience the sensation that they are going to have a "normal" bowel movement from their rectum. This sensation is known as "phantom rectum" and can be distressing for those who experience it if they are not prepared for it. They feel as if they have to pass a stool, but they know their rectum has been removed. You may have heard of people who lose limbs or fingers yet who experience a sensation as if the limb or finger were still there. This "phantom limb" phenomenon occurs because the nerves that supplied the limb are still in place, even though the limb has gone. The brain still "thinks" the limb is there. This is what happens with phantom rectum—the nerves to the rectum are still intact, even though the surgeon has removed the rectum itself. The brain "thinks" the rectum should get ready to pass a stool. Phantom rectum is a normal sensation and usually disappears as the brain gets used to the fact that waste is expelled from the ostomy and not from the rectum.

Temporary Colostomy

A colostomy may be created as only a temporary arrangement when a diseased part of the bowel has been removed, so that the remaining parts of the bowel can have time to heal. It is sometimes formed temporarily when the surgeon wants to observe how another part of the digestive system is working. A temporary colostomy might also be formed when an injury to the anus or rectum needs time to heal. With a temporary colostomy the waste material is diverted away from a part of the digestive system (e.g., the rectum or anus) to the abdomen until it is safe for the waste to pass along its usual route again. This is a bit like a road detour, where cars are diverted to another route until the old road is repaired.

The rectum is left in place when the colostomy is only a temporary arrangement. This means that the large intestine, which has been diverted to the abdomen, can be rejoined to the rectum at a later date.

Loop Colostomy

A loop colostomy is when a loop of bowel is brought to the surface of the skin and opened up. It is supported by a rod. Only one of the two openings actively produces waste material. It is almost always a temporary arrangement. The two openings can be joined again later.

Other Types of Colostomy

You may remember from Chapter 1 that by the time food reaches the large intestine, it has been transformed first into chyme (in the stomach) and then into chyle (in the small intestine); in the large intestine, water and chemicals are absorbed. The consistency of the waste material that comes out of the colostomy depends on which part of the large intestine the surgeon has diverted to the abdomen. If the surgeon diverts a piece of large intestine which is further along, that is, nearer the rectum, then the waste that comes out of the ostomy is harder than if the surgeon had diverted a piece of intestine at the beginning of the large intestine. This is because more water has been absorbed by the time the waste has reached the parts of the large intestine nearer the rectum.

The decision about which part of the large intestine to bring to the abdomen's surface depends on the position of the disease in the digestive system. Figure 1 (page 8) shows the different parts of the colon—the ascending colon, the transverse colon, the descending colon, and the sigmoid colon. You may hear the terms *transverse colostomy* or *sigmoid colostomy*. These terms define which part of the large intestine has been brought to the abdominal surface. A sigmoid colostomy, for example, is a colostomy in which the sigmoid section of the large intestine has been redirected to form a new outlet on the abdominal surface.

What Is an Ileostomy?

Ileostomy is the name given to an opening made during an operation in which the small intestine is brought to the surface of the abdomen so that waste material comes out there, instead of travelling on within the digestive system to the large intestine. An ileostomy usually comes out on the lower right side of the abdomen. The waste material that exits from this type of stoma is much more watery (a bit like porridge) than the waste that comes from a colostomy. The waste from an ileostomy contains digestive enzymes that are harmful to the skin. Because of this, an ileostomy always sticks out more than a colostomy does; this helps to keep the chemicals away from the skin as much as possible. An ileostomy is usually situated to the right of and just below the navel.

When all of the colon, rectum, and anal canal are removed and an ileostomy is formed, the procedure is called a pan procto-colectomy with ileostomy. This is always performed as a permanent arrangement. Sometimes the surgeon performs an operation called a total colectomy with ileostomy. This means that the colon is removed but the rectum stays in place. The rectum is either just left in place, or it can be diverted to the abdominal surface to form a mucus fistula. This might be done if the surgeon is thinking of performing more surgery in the future, in which case he/she needs to keep the rectum in place.

Earlier in the chapter, we learned about the procedure called loop colostomy. It is also possible to make a loop ileostomy, where a loop of small intestine is brought to the abdominal surface and fixed so that one end forms a spout. The other end is an opening that leads to the large intestine. This is usually done as a temporary arrangement; the ends can be rejoined later.

Alternatives to Ileostomy

Surgeons are always developing new techniques, and these include variations on the operations discussed above. This book does not aim to provide details on all possible surgical procedures. A surgeon is always the best source of information on these techniques and will be able to tell you which options are relevant to your particular situation. However, I have decided to include information on two increasingly popular alternatives to ileostomy surgery; these options allow patients to avoid having to wear an appliance at all times. They are called the Kock pouch and the ileo-anal pouch.

The Kock Pouch

A Kock pouch is made by creating a pouch and a small valve from the small intestine. The patient inserts a catheter through the valve to drain off the contents, usually four to five times each day. This operation is not suitable for everyone.

The Ileo-Anal Pouch

Surgery to create an ileo-anal pouch is not appropriate for conditions such as Crohn's disease. An ileo-anal pouch is a specially created pouch that holds waste material and is joined to the anus. Waste material is thus expelled from the anus as normal. This happens more frequently than normal, though (four to six times a day and once at night), and the waste material is very loose.

An ileo-anal pouch is created in stages. The first stage involves the removal of the colon and the formation of a temporary ileostomy. A pouch is then made from part of the small intestine, and this is attached to the anus. The final stage is when the temporary ileostomy is reversed, allowing the waste material to pass through the pouch. The muscles around the anus need to be strong for this operation to work. Special assessments and exercises to strengthen these muscles may be recommended. It can take longer to get used to an ileo-anal pouch than it does to get used to an ileostomy. If you think this option may be a possibility for you, discuss it with your doctor.

What Is a Urostomy?

Urostomy is the name given to an opening made during an operation in which urine is diverted to the surface of the abdomen so that it can be collected there, instead of being stored in the bladder and then passed through the urethra. Urostomies are usually performed when the bladder has to be removed (cystectomy). During the procedure, a piece of the small intestine is removed and brought to the surface of the person's abdomen. The tubes that carry urine from the kidneys (ureters) are sewn to the end of the piece of small intestine, allowing the urine to flow out of the ostomy. A urostomy is usually situated to the right of and just below the navel. It is sometimes called an ileal conduit or urinary diversion ostomy.

Two Ostomies

Sometimes people have two ostomies created. They may already have one ostomy and then need to have another one because they develop a different disease. Other people must have two ostomies made at the same time because of the nature or spread of their illness. These are created in the same way as has been described for one ostomy. Living with two ostomies can be particularly difficult, though many of the issues are the same as those which occur when someone has one ostomy—issues which this book aims to cover.

Deciding on the Position of the Ostomy

The decision about where the ostomy should come out of your abdomen is a very important one—and one in which you are involved (unless it's an emergency operation). An important consideration is that you need to be able to see the ostomy; this is helpful when it comes to looking after it. It is also important to check that the position is suitable for you whether you are sitting, standing, or lying. An ostomy-care nurse or ostomy nurse (called an enterostomal therapist, or ET, in the United States) or doctor should be involved in helping you choose a site for the ostomy. He/she works to ensure that possible sites for the ostomy will not interfere with clothing, and also takes many other things into account, such as the presence of scars, the position of the navel, creases in the groin, the waistline, fatty bulges, the place where the surgeon will make the cuts, and any areas affected by skin problems.

When you have decided with the nurse or doctor on a position for the ostomy, it will be marked with a special pen. At this stage, some people start to worry that they might not be able to wear the clothes they used to. I once saw a patient who was upset because she thought she would have to discard all her clothes. There may be individual items of clothing you feel less comfortable wearing, but there's no reason why certain garments (e.g., tight jeans) can't be worn if you wish. Having an ostomy does not mean having to buy a completely new wardrobe.

Sometimes it is necessary to have a second operation at a later date to move the ostomy slightly or to tidy it up in some way. This is referred to as refashioning the ostomy. Further operations can sometimes be necessary if you have problems—such as a prolapse (the stoma sticks out more than it should) or a retraction (the stoma falls in)—that need attention.

Summary

This chapter has explained the main types of ostomy that can be created. Some of the important factors in siting the ostomy have been outlined. You have read about the way the digestive system works, some of the problems that can arise in the digestive system, and the main ostomy operations that are carried out to treat these diseases. To show yourself that you understand what a colostomy, ileostomy, or urostomy is, you might want to try explaining them to a family member or friend.

Colostomy is the name given to the opening made during an operation in which the large intestine is brought to the surface of the abdomen. There are different versions of this operation (e.g., abdominoperineal resection and loop colostomy).

Ileostomy is the name given to the opening made during an operation in which the small intestine is brought to the surface of the abdomen. There are different versions of this operation (e.g., pan proctocolectomy and loop ileostomy).

Alternatives to ileostomy surgery exist that avoid the need to wear an ostomy appliance; the Kock pouch and ileo-anal pouch are examples of these. A surgeon should be able to advise you on these procedures.

Urostomy is the name given to the opening made during an operation in which urine is diverted to the surface of the abdomen. This is done by joining the ureters to a piece of small intestine.

The important decision about exactly where on the abdomen to site the ostomy is made before the operation, by a specially trained nurse or doctor who makes a decision based on you as an individual.

The next chapter will cover some of the main issues that are important for you to understand before undergoing an ostomy operation.

Chapter 3

What to Expect in the Hospital

This chapter provides information on various aspects of your contact with hospitals: information you may wish to have before entering the hospital, tests you might undergo, the staff you are likely to interact with there, and the surgical procedure itself. So much happens to you when you are in the hospital that it can be very difficult to remember it all. But having the information you want and being satisfied with it is an important part of beginning life with an ostomy. This chapter aims to help you with that.

My Information Needs

One of the most important factors that determines how well a person adjusts psychologically to an operation is whether they are satisfied with the information they receive. You will have your own ideas about the information you want to know before surgery. Make a list below of the questions you want answered before the operation; this way, you will not forget what you want to know, and there is a better chance of getting all your questions answered.

You will notice that some nurses and doctors make notes when they are asking you questions, to help them remember what you tell them. Similarly, to remember what *they* tell *you*, you should also write down their answers to your questions—in the spaces provided below, if you wish. You will thus have a reminder of what was said, which can be referred to later. This can be useful when you need to explain various details about your situation to others, such as relatives or friends. It can also help if you want to read it over again yourself.

Before the Operation

Examples: How long will I be in the hospital before my operation? Will any tests be carried out? What are they?

Question:

Answer:

. . . .

Question:

Answer:

. . . .

Question:

Answer:

. . . .

During the Operation

Examples: How many people will be in the operating room? What will the surgeon do if it looks worse than he/she anticipated?

Question:

Answer:

. . . .

Question:

Answer:

. . . .

Question:

Answer:

. . . .

After the Operation

Examples: Will the ostomy start working right away? How will I know if the operation has been succesful or not? Will my sexual functioning be affected?

Question:

Answer:

. . . .

Question:

Answer:

. . . .

Question:

Answer:

. . . .

Now that you have thought about what you would like to know beforehand, you can begin to check off each question as it is answered. This book may help answer some of your questions. Doctors, nurses, and other hospital staff are also important sources for information. Once you have listed all your questions, you can tell your nurse or doctor about the list and ask to work through it with them. You might be worried that the nurse or doctor will be too busy, or that you are being a nuisance. But remember that answering a patient's questions and providing information is part of their job; if you are worried about their being too busy, you can ask them to set aside time to discuss your questions later. You might be embarrassed about asking certain questions, or unsure how to go about this. There are no easy answers on how to overcome embarrassment. You might want to confide your embarrassment to a nurse or other staff member who will help you to overcome it, or you might want to ask if a friend or family member could be with you when you ask your questions.

It is important that you are as satisfied as possible with the information you get about the ostomy operation before you undergo it. This may include seeing photographs of what the ostomy will look like, or even meeting someone who has had an ostomy operation. Every person is different—there can be no hard and fast rule about what is the best thing to do. But if you have not yet undergone surgery and you think you might want to see an ostomy or to meet someone who has one, then talk this over with your health-care team. The ET will help you reach a decision about what seems to be the best option for you. If you do decide to meet someone who has had an ostomy operation, please remember that this is just one person. If you have a concern or a problem that they do not mention, this does not mean that you need to be especially worried. Everyone is different.

People who have had an ostomy for many years can be very positive about their life with an ostomy. Some patients who are awaiting their own ostomy operation undoubtedly find this very helpful. However, it can cause problems for others who imagine they will never be so positive. I am sure that if you ask the person to tell you honestly, he or she will share his or her worries with you as well. Remember that getting used to life with an ostomy is a gradual process. Even if you experience a few hiccups along the way, they can usually be sorted out and you can be helped back on track again. There are trained people who will do all they can to help you with whatever problem might develop.

Medical Tests

Certain tests are carried out by doctors to help them determine the nature of your problem and which treatment is best for you. You may already have had some of these tests—or you might have them in the future. The main medical tests people undergo before or after an ostomy operation are outlined below.

Barium Enema

A barium enema allows the X-ray examination of the large intestine. A thick, liquidy substance (barium liquid) is fed into the large intestine by means of a tube which is inserted through the anus. Barium is a substance which shows up on an X ray, enabling the doctor to spot any possible problems, such as inflammation or ulcers. Some air is also blown into the bowel to help obtain more detailed X rays.

The test is not painful, though you may feel a little uncomfortable for a short time. The test lasts for no longer than thirty minutes from beginning to end. You are given laxatives to take on the day of your appointment. If you have a morning appointment, you are asked to skip breakfast. For afternoon appointments, you are allowed to have a light breakfast before 8:00 A.M., but you must have nothing to eat or drink after this.

In some cases, barium enema tests are arranged after the ostomy operation so that the surgeon can check the bowel. In this case, the barium liquid is inserted through the ostomy.

CT Scan

A CT or computerized tomography scan is a specialized form of X-ray examination which provides pictures of internal organs not accessible to normal X-ray machines. A CT scan is carried out when the doctor wants to get pictures of certain internal parts of your body. You lie on a flat surface while the scanner rotates around you, producing images of the inside of your body. When you have a CT scan of the abdomen or pelvis, you are given a small quantity of liquid to drink about one hour before you are scanned. You should expect to be at the hospital for half an hour to two hours.

Intravenous Pyelogram (IVP) or Intravenous Urogram (IVU)

An IVP or IVU is an X ray of the kidneys and bladder. You are given a special dye containing iodine, usually by injection into a vein in your arm. The dye shows up in the various parts of the urinary system on the X ray, revealing whether there are any problems and, if so, where exactly they are.

Some people say that they feel hot and flushed when the dye is injected. But there is no pain and there are no aftereffects involved with this test. You need to follow a special diet for three days before the test. This is called a low-residue diet and includes foods such as lean meat, boiled potatoes, well-cooked root vegetables, tea, fruit juice, plain crackers, and strained soup. You are also required to take laxatives before the appointment. Previous to a morning appointment you should not eat anything, and for an afternoon appointment you should have nothing to eat or drink after a light breakfast. The test is usually finished within one hour.

Ultrasound

Ultrasound uses radio waves to look inside the body without using X rays. Ultrasound is used to look at developing babies in the womb, and it is also used in other areas of health care to examine other parts of the body. A bit of gel is applied to the skin, and a small scanner is moved over the surface of the body to take pictures of what is happening inside. The same eating restrictions apply to this test as to a barium enema (see above). You are also required to drink a pint of water or diluted juice before the ultrasound, and you must not empty your bladder beforehand. The bladder needs to be full for this test.

Sigmoidoscopy

This test is done when the doctor wants to be able to see the anus, rectum, and sigmoid colon (see Chapter 1 for discussion and illustration of these body parts). A long, flexible tube with a light on the end—called a sigmoidoscope—is inserted through the anus and rectum. The doctor can see inside the body by looking through a miniature telescope at the other end of the tube. Using this technique, it is also possible to remove a piece of the bowel to look at it carefully under a microscope; this is called a biopsy, and it is another procedure that can help your health-care team detect internal problems. A sigmoidoscopy takes a maximum of twenty to thirty minutes and may involve your being given a mild sedative.

Colonoscopy

Sometimes doctors want to see all of the large intestine (colon). A long, flexible viewing tube—called a colonoscope—is inserted into the colon through the anus and rectum. People who have this test are often given a tablet or an injection to make them sleepy. It is possible to feel the tube moving inside you during this test. As with a sigmoidoscopy, this may feel a little uncomfortable for a short time. The test is perfectly safe and lasts for a maximum of thirty minutes from beginning to end.

Cystoscopy

This test is similar to a sigmoidoscopy, but instead, the flexible tube (cystoscope) is inserted through the urethra (see Chapter 1) and then into the bladder. This helps the doctor see if there is anything wrong in the bladder. During a cystoscopy, a small piece of tissue can be removed from the bladder to be examined under a microscope.

General Information

For most of these medical tests, you will be asked to take off all your clothing and change into a gown. Most tests do not require a general anesthetic, but if one is required, you will be told about it; in such a case, the test may still be done on an outpatient basis. Perhaps you will be asked to undergo other tests that have not been mentioned here and that you are unfamiliar with—ask your nurse or doctor to explain what is involved.

If you must go for a medical test, you may feel nervous. Some people understandably get tense about going for a test and dread it from the minute they are told it is needed. Here are some things you can do to reduce your nervousness about going for a medical test.

Getting factual information about the test can be helpful. When we lack information, we tend to "fill in the blanks" by predicting that negative things will happen and that we won't be able to cope. Getting accurate information helps us to challenge these fear-based ideas. The staff in your doctor's office or at the hospital might be able to give you an information leaflet if you ask for one. You might also want to obtain answers to the following questions before you undergo a test:

* What does it involve?

* Why is it being done?

* How long will it take?

* Will it be painful?

* What might the results show?

* When will I learn the results?

If someone else you know has had the particular test done it can also help to talk to them; they might be able to tell you about what happened and how they coped with it.

On the other hand, research has shown that some people prefer not to have information. If this is what you prefer, then it may be the best option for you. The important thing is that whatever information you ask for—however small or insignificant it may seem to you—you get answers that satisfy you.

Another thing that can be helpful in coping with medical tests is to think up things to say to yourself during the test. Examples of this would be: "This is okay; I can cope with this and take it one step at a time" or "This is only for a few minutes, and it is to find out what is wrong with me" or "I can do this, no problem; I know what is happening, and this is to help me."

You might also want to keep your mind occupied while the test is going on. There are various ways in which you can do this. One way is to imagine a delightful scene and to focus on it in detail (the sights, sounds, smells, and colors) during the test. Some people picture a pleasant holiday they have enjoyed or imagine themselves in a really relaxing situation or at an enjoyable family event. Another way of distracting yourself is to play mental games: Count backward from 100 in sevens (100, 93, 86, etc.), or within one minute think of as many words as possible beginning with the letter *s*, or try to come up with the name of a town for every letter of the alphabet. Such mental distractions help to block out thoughts which might cause distress during the test. (The distraction technique may also be helpful at other times when you want a quick way of coping with anxious or worrisome thoughts.)

Who's Who at the Hospital

In the course of your contact with the hospital, you will meet many different health professionals. It can be confusing to meet so many different people with different jobs and sometimes obscure titles. The following list covers the staff whom you are most likely to meet when you are in the hospital. There may be other health professionals who are involved in your care; if you do not know who they are or what they do, ask them to tell you.

Resident

A resident is a fully qualified medical doctor who is gaining more experience in a specific area of medicine or surgery—in other words, you might meet a resident in surgery or a resident in general medicine. Residents are involved in arranging tests, assessing symptoms, and recommending treatments. The term "intern" used to be used to refer to a doctor gaining experience in the first year following qualification. A chief resident is a resident in his/her last year of training who takes on administrative functions for the residency training program such as scheduling or teaching.

Fellow

"Fellows" are doctors who have completed specialized training and taken further exams in one particular area of medicine, beyond the requirements for eligibility for initial certification in their chosen area of medical practice. They have overall responsibility for some of the patients they see and may eventually become chiefs. A Fellow in surgery may actually perform your ostomy operation.

Attending Physician

An attending physician is a fully trained senior doctor who has responsibility for a particular area of medical care within a hospital—such as surgery, urology, or medicine. An attending physician is usually directly involved in planning your treatment with you—for example, in deciding what tests to order and what treatments to recommend.

Oncologist

An oncologist is a doctor who specializes in the diagnosis and treatment of cancers.

Urologist

A urologist is a doctor who specializes in the diagnosis and treatment of problems associated with the urinary system.

Enterostomal Therapist (ET)

The enterostomal therapist (commonly called the ET) is a specialist nurse who has been trained in the care of people before and after ostomy surgery. The ET has special expertise in all aspects of ostomy care, including teaching patients to look after their ostomy, giving information and advice, supporting patients, helping with ostomy-care routines, and advising on problems such as leakage. The ET is the main person who helps the patient before and after the ostomy operation.

Occupational Therapist (OT)

OTs are health-care professionals with special expertise in advising on daily living activities, such as cooking and dressing. They might help someone who is having these practical problems by advising on new ways of dealing with the activities or by providing aids to help make the activities easier. You might come across an OT if you have this type of problem after having an ostomy formed.

Physical Therapist

Physical therapists are skilled in helping patients to become active as soon as possible after an operation. Difficulty with movement can be common after an ostomy operation—and the resulting inactivity can mean an increased risk of infections and other problems. The physical therapist usually visits before an operation to explain the therapy program and may also teach you some simple breathing and movement exercises.

Clinical Psychologist

Clinical psychologists are specialists in the way people feel, think, and behave. They have expertise in the psychological aspects of physical and mental health and are trained to carry out psychological assessments and treat people to enable them to overcome problems with their feelings, thoughts, and/or behavior. Ostomy patients might see a clinical psychologist if they develop problems with anxiety or depression, or develop sexual problems after surgery.

Dietician

Dieticians have special expertise in the science of nutrition, and they use their knowledge to promote nutritional well-being, to treat disease, and to prevent nutrition-related problems. Ostomy patients usually receive advice on diet from their ET, but a dietician may be involved if specific nutritional problems develop. Dieticians will assess your diet history and gather information on your weight, including any changes.

The Operation...and Immediately After

Before you undergo the operation to make an ostomy, you will have to make sure that your bowel is as clear of food and waste material as possible. This is called bowel preparation. It can be done in different ways; you will have to stop eating the day before the operation, and you might be given an enema or some laxative tablets. An enema is a medicine that is inserted up your anus and makes you want to empty the contents of your bowel. Its purpose is to make the bowel as clean as possible, so that the bowel is easier to see during tests. More importantly, an empty bowel creates less chance of an infection developing in the bowel after surgery.

After the operation you will probably have tubes and IVs going into your body. Some of the tubes are to make sure that fluids and drugs get into your body; others help rid your body of fluids and waste material. You will probably have a tube, called a nasogastric tube, inserted into your nose. It travels down your esophagus and into your stomach. It will probably remain in place until your body starts to recover from the operation and works as it is supposed to.

You will probably wait a couple of days before looking at your ostomy. The ostomy will be much much bigger at first than it will be in a few weeks. It will get smaller as each day passes, usually settling at about an inch or an inch and a quarter in diameter.

If you have had a colostomy or ileostomy, you will notice that there is no waste material produced for a few days. This is normal. You will also notice a foul smell when the bag is changed for the first time. Just as the ostomy is much bigger at first, so is the smell worse in the early days. This is because your bowel has not been working for some days. There has been a buildup of bacteria inside, and this is what creates the foul odor. Unlike a colostomy or an ileostomy, a urostomy starts to work almost immediately after the operation.

Summary

Being satisfied with the advance information you receive about both the operation and the ostomy is an important part of beginning life with an ostomy.

You might have to undergo medical tests, such as a barium enema, CT scan, intravenous pyelogram, sigmoidoscopy, or cystoscopy. Understanding what will happen during these tests can make them easier to cope with. Additionally, a number of practical ways exist whereby you can reduce anxiety before the tests and make the tests themselves easier to cope with.

The many different hospital staffers can be confusing. Don't be afraid to ask them what their jobs are and why, specifically, they are seeing you!

Before the ostomy operation, some people want to look at a picture of an ostomy or talk to someone who has had an ostomy operation. Think about whether you would find this helpful.

An ostomy is much bigger and much smellier just after the operation than it will be in the days and weeks afterwards.

The ET is there to help you learn how to look after the ostomy and will make sure you can do this before you go home. Learning how to look after the ostomy means that you need to learn about ostomy-care appliances—"bags" or "pouches." The next chapter outlines the different types of appliances and helps you think about your ostomy-care routine and how to incorporate it into your everyday life. It is important that you be confident about looking after your ostomy before you go home. The next chapter includes a diary to help you to keep track of your progress in caring for the ostomy.

Chapter 4

The Ostomy-Care Routine

Before I left the hospital, most of the self-pity I'd felt had been erased by learning from the experience of others. I was introduced by the ostomy nurse to different appliances and was taught how to change the bag and clean the area. By the time I was discharged, I was using a one-piece disposable bag, feeling positive, and was supplied with a purpose-filled "box of tricks."

Male colostomy patient, age 63

When you have an ostomy operation, not only do you need to get used to life with an ostomy, you also need to get used to life with ostomy-care appliances. People have different preferences about what they call their ostomy-care appliance—some people call it a bag, whereas others prefer to call it a pouch. I will refer to it as an appliance in this chapter. The ostomy appliance is a device specially manufactured to collect the waste material produced from the ostomy. After you have had an ostomy operation, you need to learn what is involved with your new routine for getting rid of waste. This means learning a new set of skills and becoming familiar with a new set of words to describe the various parts of the ostomy appliance and the tasks associated with changing it. Eventually the new routine becomes a habit— just like the old habits involved with the disposing of waste before the ostomy operation.

Ostomy-Care Appliances

Ostomy-care appliances come in either one or two pieces.

The *one-piece appliance* has a bag to collect waste material (this has a hole in it that fits neatly around the ostomy) and an outer ring. This outer ring, called a flange, is adhesive and sticks securely to your skin to keep the appliance in place. You can buy appliances with holes already cut to the size of your ostomy (most manufacturers provide guides to measure ostomy sizes). Alternatively, you can buy appliances which do not have holes cut in them and then cut the hole in the flange to fit your ostomy exactly. All of a one-piece appliance—the bag and the outer ring—is disposed of when the bag is full of waste material. The whole thing (bag and outer ring) is then replaced with a completely new appliance. (A section on the disposal of ostomy-care appliances appears later in the chapter.)

The *two-piece appliance* has a base plate that fits around the ostomy. The base plate is fitted with adhesive material to make it stick to your skin. The second part of the two-piece appliance is the bag that fixes on to the base plate. Unlike a one-piece appliance, only the bag is disposed of. The plate does not need to be removed each time you change the bag; it can stay in place and a new bag can be clipped on when you have disposed of the old one.

Ostomy-care appliances can be drainable or closed.

A *drainable ostomy-care appliance* can be opened at one end so that the contents can be emptied or drained away. Drainable appliances are usually used by people who have an ileostomy. Sometimes they may also be used immediately after a colostomy operation, when the waste material is very liquid and it is easier to drain the contents. You may remember from Chapter 2 that the waste material from an ileostomy is loose in consistency; therefore, a drainable appliance makes emptying easier.

Closed ostomy-care appliances do not have an opening at the end. They are therefore better suited to use when the waste material is more solid, as with most colostomies.

Ostomy-care appliances can be either transparent or opaque. The transparent (see-through) appliance is helpful when you want to be able to see the ostomy and the waste material. This may be important in the early stages following your operation; it will help you to see the ostomy while you are getting used to all that is involved with the ostomy-care routine. Additionally, it may be helpful for you or your doctor to see the waste material. Your doctor might observe the color and/or consistency to check on your progress. Getting the appliance into the correct position over the ostomy can be easier with a transparent appliance. When you do not need or want to see the ostomy or the waste material, there are opaque appliances that have a pattern or a tint on them.

There are various combinations of ostomy-care appliance available: one-piece closed opaque, two-piece closed opaque, one-piece drainable transparent, etc. Now that you know what each of these terms means, you can appreciate what makes each of these appliances different. Learning about ostomy-care appliances is a bit like having to learn to use a new language.

Urostomy appliances are slightly different from the appliances used most commonly for colostomies and ileostomies. Because urine is produced much more frequently than fecal waste, the appliances used for urostomies are designed to be worn for longer periods. Urostomy appliances have a drainage tap and valve to prevent the urine from travelling back up near the ostomy when the patient is lying down. This is very important, because it reduces the chances of infection. The rest of the appliance for a urostomy is similar to those used for colostomies and ileostomies.

Most people with a urostomy will have to use a night drainage system when they are asleep. This means that the urine is being collected in a larger pouch overnight. The pouch is fixed to a stand. If you have a urostomy and are worried that the pouch might leak, the stand for the night drainage bag can be placed in a basin—so if there is a leak, it goes into the bowl and not onto the carpet.

There have been many advances since the days of the first ostomy-care appliances. I have read many stories of people who had to use things like thick, black rubber bags for collecting waste from an ostomy—and even of people having to improvise using a baked-bean can. Most colostomy and ileostomy bags nowadays are fitted with a special carbon filter that deodorizes (takes the smell away from) the gases that can come from the ostomy. Appliances are made of materials that are odor-proof and make little noise when you move. The flange is made of a special material that is designed not to irritate your skin.

Changing the Appliance

Learning to change the ostomy-care appliance is an important part of adjusting to life with an ostomy. Initially, you may think that it will never become "routine," that you will never have confidence or get used to what is involved. This may or may not be true—you will learn for yourself as time goes on. Women patients might find it helpful to think back to when they first learned to deal with the hygiene routine associated with menstruation. Did you have doubts that you would be able to get used to it? Were you superconfident about inserting a tampon or using a sanitary pad on the first few occasions? You probably had doubts and were not very confident to start with. And you almost certainly became more confident as time went on. Changing the ostomy appliance is the same—you probably will have some doubts to start with, but with time it will become easier as your confidence increases.

Male patients might also compare the situation with things they weren't confident about to begin with—for example, being afraid of cutting yourself the first time you used a razor or feeling uncertain about learning to change the tire on a car. If you think about how you felt the first time you did these things and compare then with now, you will notice that you have fewer doubts and more confidence as time goes on.

You will no doubt develop your own particular routine for changing the ostomy appliance. However, there are some basic steps you must take to change the appliance safely. One of the most important things to note is that most appliances *are not* designed to be flushed down the toilet, as this would cause a serious blockage in the plumbing.

Finally, it may be a good idea to make sure someone else in your life can change your appliance as well—a spouse, family member, or friend—just in case something happens that prevents you from doing it yourself. Some people with an ostomy find it reassuring to know that someone else is able to change the appliance if they are unable to do so.

Some people are not sure when to change their appliance. There are no hard and fast rules about this, and with time you will find out what works best for you. However, it is generally not a good idea to wait until the appliance is almost overflowing with waste material before you change it. You will get into a routine eventually.

There are certain items that you need every time you change the appliance. Some people find it helpful to collect these and to put them into a little box or bag to keep them together. Some people have two sets: one that stays at home and the other to take out as a portable ostomy-care tool set.

Each time you change the appliance, you will need the following items:

* new appliance

* measuring guide

* paper towels or wipes

* paper bag, plastic bag, or newspaper

* small pair of scissors

* small mirror

Once you have all of these items, you are ready to begin. The following steps are the main ones you will go through each time you change the appliance:

1. Locate and lay out all the items that you will need for changing the appliance.

2. Take off the old appliance.

3. Empty the contents of the old appliance into the toilet. If you have a closed appliance, this is done by cutting it with a pair of scissors. A drainable appliance can be drained into the toilet. Rinse the appliance by holding it under the flush of the toilet. You can avoid splashing from the toilet bowl by placing a couple of sheets of toilet paper or paper towels on the surface of the water before emptying the appliance contents.

4. Wrap the old appliance in newspaper or put it into a plastic bag.

5. Wipe around your ostomy with a piece of paper towel or a wipe, and then wash around the ostomy with warm water.

6. Pat the area around the ostomy dry with a piece of paper towel or toilet paper.

7. If you use any accessories (e.g., creams), they should be applied at this stage.

8. If you need to cut the pouch to size, use the measuring guide. Put on the new appliance (using the mirror may help if it is difficult to see the stoma). If it is a two-piece appliance, start with the base plate first. With urostomy bags, remember to make sure that the tap is closed. With ileostomy bags, remember to make sure the clip is tightened.

9. The old appliance (wrapped and placed in a bag) can now be placed in the trash.

You may find it helpful to use a safety pin to pin your clothing up and out of the way when you are changing the appliance.

Measuring Your Confidence: A Checklist

To help you see your increasing confidence in caring for your ostomy, I suggest that you rate your self-confidence in performing each of the main tasks at four different stages:

1. After you have tried the main steps in the ostomy-care routine before leaving the hospital

2. After one week at home

3. After one month at home

4. After three months at home

You can rate your confidence by using a scale of zero to ten for each of the tasks. A score of zero means you are not confident at all at that task, whereas a score of ten means you could not be more confident in your ability to carry out that task.

Stage 1 Rating

Date: . . . .   At the hospital ... at home (circle one)

Removing the appliance from my skin (0–10)   . . . .
Emptying the used appliance (0–10)   . . . .
Washing and drying the ostomy and skin (0–10)   . . . .
Measuring the ostomy (0–10)   . . . .
Putting on the new appliance (0–10)   . . . .
Getting rid of the used appliance (0–10)   . . . .

Stage 2 Rating

Date: . . . .   At the hospital ... at home (circle one)

Removing the appliance from my skin (0–10)   . . . .
Emptying the used appliance (0–10)   . . . .
Washing and drying the ostomy and skin (0–10)   . . . .
Measuring the ostomy (0–10)   . . . .
Putting on the new appliance (0–10)   . . . .
Getting rid of the used appliance (0–10)   . . . .

Stage 3 Rating

Date: . . . .   At the hospital ... at home (circle one)

Removing the appliance from my skin (0–10)   . . . .
Emptying the used appliance (0–10)   . . . .
Washing and drying the ostomy and skin (0–10)   . . . .
Measuring the ostomy (0–10)   . . . .
Putting on the new appliance (0–10)   . . . .
Getting rid of the used appliance (0–10)   . . . .

Stage 4 Rating

Date: . . . .   At the hospital ... at home (circle one)

Removing the appliance from my skin (0–10)   . . . .
Emptying the used appliance (0–10)   . . . .
Washing and drying ostomy and skin (0–10)   . . . .
Measuring the ostomy (0–10)   . . . .
Putting on the new appliance (0–10)   . . . .
Getting rid of the used appliance (0–10)   . . . .

When you have rated these activities on four different occasions, check to see if your confidence ratings are staying the same, getting worse, or improving. If they are not getting any better, you may want to consult with your ET. It may be that there is a problem which is making you less confident about the ostomy-care routine. The nurse will be able to help with this. If you notice that your confidence is increasing, then you might want to think about how this relates to your previous doubts that you would never learn to do the various tasks. This will be a helpful exercise should you ever try to read into the future—as you did when you first had the ostomy.

New Developments in Appliance Disposal

Disposing of an ostomy-care appliance is not the easiest thing in the world. It involves having to spend longer in the bathroom than you did before your ostomy operation, having closer contact with your own bodily waste material, and having to carry all sorts of extra items into the bathroom. Recent developments in stoma care aim to make appliance disposal a more "normal" experience. Developments in scientific technology have meant that some used appliances can now be flushed straight down the toilet—the bags are strong enough to contain the waste material when they are being worn (even during swimming), but they gradually disintegrate into biodegradable products when they are flushed down the toilet. At the time of writing, these disposable bags are only available to people with a colostomy, but scientists are working on developing similar appliances for use with ileostomies. Information on appliance manufacturers can be found in "Resources," at the end of the book.

Getting Supplies

Before you leave the hospital, you should be given the details about the appliances you have been using. You will thus know what to get when you need fresh supplies. Space is available below for you to write in this information. If you have not yet received this information, you should ask your nurse or doctor for it:

Appliance type: . . . .
Appliance manufacturer: . . . .
Appliance model: . . . .
Code/model number: . . . .
Number in pack: . . . .
Monthly quantity: . . . .

Ostomy-care appliances are issued by prescription. In other words, to obtain your ostomy-care appliances you need to get a prescription from your doctor, go to the pharmacist, and purchase the items—in the same way you would fill a prescription for pills or other medicines. Most health-insurance plans cover ostomy-care appliances.

Testing Different Appliances

In the early stages of life with an ostomy, you may try various appliances—either because you experience problems with some or because you become aware of new appliances you want to try. Different appliances suit different people. Use the pages below to note the appliances you try, your ratings for them (in the areas of comfort, confidence, and ease of change and disposal), and any other comments you may have about them. Once again, use ratings of zero to ten; if you are rating an appliance for comfort, a score of zero would mean not at all comfortable, while ten would mean the most comfortable appliance you could imagine.

Trial period: *From* . . . . *to* . . . .

    Appliance manufacturer: . . . .

    Appliance model: . . . .

    Comfort (0–10):   . . . .

    Confidence (0–10):   . . . .

    Ease of change and disposal (0–10):   . . . .

    Comments: . . . .

        . . . .

        . . . .

        . . . .

Trial period: *From* . . . . *to* . . . .

    Appliance manufacturer: . . . .

    Appliance model: . . . .

    Comfort (0–10):   . . . .

    Confidence (0–10):   . . . .

    Ease of change and disposal (0–10):   . . . .

    Comments: . . . .

        . . . .

        . . . .

        . . . .

Trial period: *From* . . . . *to* . . . .

Appliance manufacturer: . . . .

Appliance model: . . . .

Comfort (0–10): . . . .

Confidence (0–10): . . . .

Ease of change and disposal (0–10): . . . .

Comments: . . . .

. . . .

. . . .

Trial period: *From* . . . . *to* . . . .

Appliance manufacturer: . . . .

Appliance model: . . . .

Comfort (0–10): . . . .

Confidence (0–10): . . . .

Ease of change and disposal (0–10): . . . .

Comments: . . . .

. . . .

. . . .

Rating each appliance you try can be a good way of deciding which one is best for you. Keep a record of your ratings and refer back to them when you want to compare your old appliance with any new ones that become available.

Leaks

At some point the ostomy appliance may develop leaks. This can be very difficult to cope with, causing embarrassment and anxiety about going out. Ostomy-related physical problems, like leaks, have also been shown to be associated with psychological difficulties such as anxiety and depression. If you keep experiencing leaks, contact your ET or doctor to have this problem checked. There may be something they can do to stop the leakage.

Below is a list of some common reasons why leaks may occur, along with suggested solutions to the problem. You may be able to help stop your leaks by making the suggested adjustments.

Leakage Troubleshooting Guide

Appliance is not sticking to the skin properly

Make sure that the skin around the ostomy is very dry. Once you've stuck the appliance to the skin, hold your hand over the ostomy and appliance for sixty seconds to warm it and to ensure that you have the best seal possible.

Folds or creases in the skin are getting in the way

You can get special pastes to fill in the cracks (a bit like spackle for humans). This makes the surface flatter and thus easier to stick the appliance onto. Speak to your ET if you need help or advice about this.

Skin around the ostomy is irritated

This can be difficult, as you can get stuck in a vicious cycle (especially with an ileostomy) whereby you have a leak that irritates the skin, which in turn prevents the appliance from adhering well. The best solution for this is to try to keep the skin around the ostomy as healthy as possible. If necessary, pay a visit to your family doctor or to a dermatologist to get treatment for your skin.

The appliance is not emptied often enough

Overfilling the appliance can break the seal because of the weight of the waste materials. Try to empty the appliance before it becomes too heavy. This stops it from pulling on the sticky seal.

High temperatures are affecting the materials of the flange

Try changing the appliance more frequently in warm weather, and/or experiment with a change of flange material.

Appliance is stored improperly or for too long

Ostomy-care appliances do not last forever. They should always be stored in a cool, dry place. You may want to ascertain from the appliance manufacturer how long they can be kept.

Alternatives

There are sometimes alternatives to wearing an ostomy-care appliance full-time. People with a colostomy may be able to use a soft foam plug that fits into the ostomy, so there is no need to wear an appliance at all times. However, they must wear an appliance at some point to collect waste material. It is also possible to use a technique called irrigation. This involves introducing flowing water into the bowel from the ostomy to ensure that waste material is expelled. Irrigation enables the person with a colostomy to have more control over their bowel movements. More information on plugs and irrigation can be obtained from your ET.

Summary

Getting used to life with an ostomy also involves getting used to ostomy-care appliances—what they are and how to change them.

Ostomy-care appliances can be one-piece or two-piece, closed or drainable, and transparent or opaque.

Changing an ostomy-care appliance can be difficult at first, but like anything new it becomes easier with practice. Your doubts will disappear and your confidence will increase.

There are many different kinds of ostomy-care appliances— trying different types and makes of appliances is often the only way to discover which one is the best for you.

Leaks can occur sometimes. They are often associated with common problems that can be easily addressed.

Plug or irrigation techniques are alternatives for some patients who prefer these to wearing a colostomy appliance full-time.

Chapter 5

Thoughts About Your Ostomy

The way we think about things is extremely important in determining how we feel, what we do, and what physical reactions we have. Events or situations do not cause our feelings—rather, our feelings come from the thoughts we have about events or situations. Similarly, events don't cause our behavior; it is the thoughts we have about the events that cause our behavior. This is important in trying to understand the different emotional, behavioral, and physical reactions of people who have undergone an ostomy operation.

To see the importance of thoughts in our everyday lives, consider this example. As you are sitting reading this book on getting used to life with an ostomy

1. You think: "This book is really interesting and has some good ideas to help me."

   * How do you think you might feel if you thought this? (circle one of the responses below)

     Depressed   Enthusiastic   Frustrated   Happy

   * What do you think you might do if you thought this? (circle one of the responses below)

     Return book to shop   Stop reading it   Keep reading it

2. You think: "This book is boring—I have wasted my money and could have bought something else more useful."

   ✳ How do you think you might feel if you thought this instead? (circle one of the responses below)

   Depressed   Enthusiastic   Frustrated   Happy

   ✳ What do you think you might do if you thought this? (circle one of the responses below)

   Return book to shop   Stop reading it   Keep reading it

3. You think: "I don't understand any of this—I am so hopeless, nothing ever goes right for me."

   ✳ How do you think you might feel if you thought this instead? (circle one of the responses below)

   Depressed   Enthusiastic   Frustrated   Happy

   ✳ What do you think you might do if you thought this? (circle one of the responses below)

   Return book to shop   Stop reading it   Keep reading it

You will notice that you had different feelings and different actions depending on your thoughts about the situation. The situation stayed exactly the same (sitting reading this book). But your thoughts were different each time, so your feelings and behaviors were also different.

In exactly the same way, it is your thoughts about the ostomy that determine your feelings and behavior toward the ostomy after the operation. Your thoughts about the ostomy determine whether you feel anxious, contented, or gloomy about it and whether you will behave similarly to the way you always have or whether you will develop new and different reactions, such as avoiding meeting new people.

There are common themes in the thought patterns of people who have had an ostomy operation. I have carried out research in this area and have listed below some of the thoughts typically experienced by people with an ostomy. To find out whether you have these thoughts, circle the word "agree" or "disagree" beside each ostomy-related thought. Try to answer each question as honestly as you can—this in itself may help you recognize some of the negative thought patterns you hold about your ostomy.

1. My ostomy rules my life.   *Agree   Disagree*
2. No one can tell that I have an ostomy.   *Agree   Disagree*
3. I am less confident in myself since I   *Agree   Disagree*
   have an ostomy.
4. No one understands what it is like to   *Agree   Disagree*
   have an ostomy.
5. I smell because of my ostomy.   *Agree   Disagree*
6. I can take part in the same activities I *Agree   Disagree*
   used to, despite my ostomy.
7. I feel less like a real man/woman since *Agree   Disagree*
   my ostomy operation.
8. I feel in control of my body following   *Agree   Disagree*
   my ostomy operation.
9. My ostomy might leak if I go out.   *Agree   Disagree*
10. I can be near other people without   *Agree   Disagree*
    worrying about my ostomy.
11. My ostomy is repulsive.   *Agree   Disagree*
12. Other people can see my bag through *Agree   Disagree*
    my clothes.
13. I am still a complete person despite   *Agree   Disagree*
    my ostomy.

The rest of this chapter focuses on these common thought patterns regarding an ostomy. It shows you how to step back from negative ostomy-related thoughts and begin to modify them. This is important in helping you to overcome negative feelings, such as anxiety or depression, about your ostomy. Changing your thinking about the ostomy is also important in changing your behavior related to it. (The next chapter includes additional, detailed information on how to identify negative thought patterns and problem thoughts and how you can then begin to modify them to help you feel better.)

Altering Negative Thought Patterns

It can be challenging to modify thought patterns, because often they're so ingrained in our mind that we fail to even realize we're carrying them. The first step is to recognize the thoughts you have about something. Doing so requires a little digging, and this section aims to help you with that.

The following sections are based on answers to the questionnaire above and are designed to help you recognize and then modify your thinking about having an ostomy. Each section heading describes a typical thought pattern; beneath it appear the related questionnaire statements and answers ("agree" or "disagree") that show negative thought patterns. The rest of the section then examines and challenges the assumptions behind the negative thought pattern.

"I'm not in control anymore."

Question 1: My ostomy rules my life.   *Agree*

Question 8: I feel in control of my body following my ostomy operation.   *Disagree*

If you believe that your ostomy rules your life or that you are no longer in control of your body, you are likely to feel sad, gloomy, or even depressed. Ask yourself: "In what way does my ostomy rule my life? Does it rule my life twenty-four hours a day, seven days a week—or just part of the time?"

Is it helpful to use the word *rules*—or is this a bit extreme? Would it be more helpful to say to yourself that the ostomy only affects how you live your life, not that it rules your life? If you think about it, most people have something or another that affects how they live their lives. Most of us have to take at least a number of different factors into account when planning our lives—and an ostomy can be thought of as another factor that needs to be taken into account. If the ostomy only affects your life during part of the week, then you can make a plan to work around this and to get on with your life at other times. One way of doing this is to keep a weekly diary of how your ostomy influences your life and then to use this information to plan your life around it. You do not have control over when your ostomy is working—that is a fact. Does this mean that you are not in control of your body? Were you always in control of your body before the ostomy operation? Did you ever have the experience of your stomach rumbling when you were with other people? Were you in control of your body then? You may not have control over when the ostomy works, but you can develop control over what effect this will have on you. You don't have control over when you will get a headache, but you can learn to cope with this by developing some control—such as taking a tablet, relaxing, or having a snooze. Does having *less* control mean that you have *none* whatsoever?

Thinking of control as something which is completely present or completely absent is not likely to be helpful. Would it help you to think in terms of having degrees of control? Some days, at certain times of the day, you may have 60 percent control—whereas, at other times you will have different amounts of control. The ostomy can only rule your life, and take away your own control, if you let it.

"Everyone knows about my ostomy."

Question 2: No one can tell that I have an ostomy.

Disagree

Question 10: I can be near other people without worrying about my ostomy.   *Disagree*

Question 12: Other people can see my bag through my
clothes.   *Agree*

If you think that people can tell you have had an ostomy operation, ask yourself *how* other people know about it. They may
know because you have mentioned it to them or because they
have heard from someone else. If this is the case, then what about
this is a problem for you? You may be worried that they will think
negatively about you because they know about your ostomy. But if
you heard that someone you knew had an ostomy, would you
think negatively of them? I suspect that you wouldn't. If you
wouldn't think negatively about someone with an ostomy, how
likely is it that people will think negatively about you? Are the
people you know really so different from you?

You may be worried about complete strangers knowing that
you have had an ostomy operation. If you are, then think carefully
about how they could possibly know about it. You might be worried that other people can tell you have an ostomy because they
see a bulge in your tummy or hear an unexpected noise. Even if
they do notice a slight bulge on your tummy (though this is unlikely unless someone is looking right at that one part of you for a
long period of time), how do you know that they would think it
was an ostomy? How many people know what an ostomy is anyway? Most people who are troubled by this thought overestimate
the degree to which other people are aware of the ostomy. They
also behave as if they can read minds—as if they know what other
people think about them. To show yourself how difficult it is to
detect an ostomy, try to pick out five people with an ostomy the
next time you spend a day out. Remember that thousands of people have ostomies—so if they are that obvious, then you should be
able to pick out a few. If you are unable to do this, perhaps it will
help you to think again about how easy it is to identify someone
with an ostomy by just looking at them. One of my patients said
that having an ostomy was like having a run in her stocking—she
knew it was there, but nobody else did.

"It's impossible for anyone to understand."

Question 4: No one understands what it is like to have an
ostomy.   *Agree*

Although you may think that no one understands, how can
this be true? Many other people have had ostomy operations—and
even if they can't understand everything that you are experiencing, is it possible that they understand most of what is happening
to you? Or perhaps they understand part of what you have been
through, and that is a start. Some people have had major operations, so they probably know something of what you have experienced. Others may know people who have ostomies. Most people
can piece together different parts of their life experience to try to
understand what you are going through.

You may be thinking that friends, family, and other people you
know don't understand what it is like to live with an ostomy—
since they don't have one, it's therefore difficult for them really to
know how it feels. But to understand something, do you have to
have experienced it yourself? Is it possible never to have experienced something, yet still to understand some of what it might be
like? Is it possible, for example, for you to understand what it
might feel like to be blind? If you close your eyes, you might get
some idea. In other words, even though you are not blind, you can
imagine and understand part of what it might be like not to see.

It is true that some people won't understand everything about
your life with an ostomy, but they may be able to imagine some of
it and to understand part of your experience by drawing on their
own experiences and those of other people. Is this good enough? If
you don't understand something, does it help you when someone
else explains it? If so, do you think it might be easier for other people to fully understand your situation if you were to give them an
explanation? You will never find out unless you try to explain and
then ask them if it has helped them in any way to understand. In
any case, do other people really need to understand fully?

"*I'm smelly.*"

Question 5: I smell because of my ostomy.   *Agree*

Is it really true to say that it is you who smells because of the ostomy? Isn't it the waste material that smells? There is a difference. You may think that other people can smell the urine or feces produced by the ostomy, and this thought may make you feel depressed or anxious. But remember that your nose is right above the ostomy, so any smell is stronger to you than it is to other people who are farther away (and whose noses are not directly above it). There may be a horrible smell when you have to empty the appliance in the bathroom—but is this really different from everyone else? The smell I produce in the bathroom, without an ostomy, is sometimes quite revolting (as my family will tell you). Telling yourself that it is you who smells doesn't help you to feel good about yourself. Perhaps you would feel better if you could remind yourself that it is the waste material that smells, not you. You might also remind yourself that all modern appliances are made of odor-proof materials.

"*I can't do the things I used to.*"

Question 3: I am less confident in myself since I have an ostomy.   *Agree*

Question 6: I can take part in the same activities I used to, despite my ostomy.   *Disagree*

Immediately after the operation there are certain things you won't be able to do, usually as a result of your having had major surgery. Does the fact that you are unable to do them now mean that you will never be able to do them again? Has there ever been a time in your life when you have been unable to do something for a while, but later you could do it again? If this has happened before, is it possible that it could happen again? When you started the activity again, did you start from where you left off or did it take some time to gradually build up to where you were? Might it be the same with the ostomy—that at first you can't do all the things you used to, but that as you recover you will be able to pick up some things, gradually working back to your old routine?

The key to dealing with this thought is to consider the things you *can* still do and to make a note of the new things you can do on each new day—for example, you might notice that you can walk longer distances. Keeping a diary is a good way of noting your gradual progress. You could start this now: Jot down two things you do each day that are new activities or activities you feel are easier than they were yesterday or the day before.

"I'm not a complete person anymore."

Question 7: I feel less like a real man/woman since my ostomy operation.   *Agree*

Question 13: I am still a complete person despite my ostomy.   *Disagree*

Some of the main concerns and problems in this area are covered in Chapter 8. But for now, consider what you would have said before the ostomy operation if someone had asked you to define what makes a real man or a real woman. Indicate below how you think you would have answered this question.

Would you have said you were a real man or woman and a complete person before the ostomy?

I would have said I was a real man/woman before the operation.   *Yes/No*

I would have said I was a complete person before the operation.   *Yes/No*

If you answered yes to one or both of these questions, you can use the exercise below. If you answered no to these questions, you may want to discuss your views with your nurse or doctor.

Before the operation, I would have said that the following things were what made me a real man/woman (it is

important to try to imagine how you would have
answered this question before the operation):

1. ....

2. ....

3. ....

Before the operation, I would have said that the following
things were what made me a complete person (it is important to try to imagine how you would have answered this
question before the operation):

1. ....

2. ....

3. ....

It will be helpful to look at your lists and see how many things
have really changed by comparing them with how things are for
you now. Have things changed as much as you thought? Have you
lost any or all of the characteristics which you would have said
made you a real man/woman or a complete person? Most people
who do this exercise can see that they have been focusing on the
one thing that is different and that it has been difficult to remember that there are other things that make you what you are and
which haven't changed. If most of the characteristics have not
changed, might it be that it is only your *thoughts* which have
changed? Perhaps you have only been focusing on the changes
since the operation and not on the things which haven't changed.
Perhaps this is making you think negatively about yourself.

Most people find, when they think carefully about these
thoughts, that they still have nearly all of the characteristics that
made them what they thought defined a "real" man or woman, or
a "complete" person. They realize that they were not thinking
about these other factors and that thinking only about the
changes was part of the problem. If, on the other hand, you have

lost some of the characteristics from your definitions, ask yourself whether they are lost forever. Is it possible that these changes are temporary and that there will be more change in the future? You may feel less like a man or a woman—but does this really mean that you *are* less of a real man or woman? Have you ever felt that something would never work out, only to find that it actually did? How we feel about something is not always necessarily the case; it can be easy to confuse feelings with facts.

"I'm afraid of leakage."

Question 9: My ostomy might leak if I go out.   *Agree*

When you go out, you might fall and break your leg accidentally—but this doesn't usually stop you from going out. There are things that you do to reduce the risk of such a thing happening—for example, you take care where and how you are walking. And, if it did happen, there are things you can do to get help or cope with it. Anxiety about leakage can stop you from going out at all. It is true that the ostomy might leak if you go out—in the same way that you might break your leg if you go out. Does focusing on this possibility help you to feel confident about going out? Would you feel confident about going for a walk if you were to dwell on the thought that you might break your leg?

There are things you can do to minimize the risk of a leak—such as making sure that your appliance is secure (see the leakage troubleshooting guide in the preceding chapter). You can also think of a coping plan that you can put into action if necessary. If the ostomy did leak, what is the worst thing that could happen? You might feel very embarrassed, but you would get cleaned up, people would understand, and life would go on. It might help to think about what you could do to cope if you noticed you were having a leak. Remember, no one ever died of embarrassment. Have you ever been embarrassed before in life? Did it feel awkward at the time? Did you cope with it? Did it pass? Did life go on? Perhaps reminding yourself of this experience will make it easier for you to cope with worries about leaks.

"It's revolting."

Question 11: My ostomy is repulsive.   *Agree*

This may be true. Again, does it really make you any different from the majority of normal human beings? Most of us have a part of our bodies which, at some time or other, we think is repulsive. If you often think this, and if it makes you feel very low in your spirits, then it may be a sign that you are having problems in coming to terms with your ostomy. You should discuss this with your ET or doctor. Perhaps you only get this thought at particular times—such as when you are changing the appliance. Think of things you could do to distract yourself as a way of taking your mind off it—like imagining what you're going to do when you have finished changing it.

If your thoughts about the ostomy are mostly negative, even after reading about different ways of thinking about it or after trying to change your thoughts, this might be a sign that you are finding it difficult to get used to life with an ostomy. It is important that you mention this to your doctor or ET so that together you can discuss ways for you to get help with this. One kind of treatment—called cognitive therapy—can be helpful for anxiety and depression caused by negative thought patterns. It helps you to identify the negative thoughts that are maintaining and feeding the anxiety and depression and thus helps you to learn ways of modifying the thoughts to make your thinking more balanced. This approach is used in the next chapter, which also includes information on common emotional reactions to ostomy surgery.

Summary

The way in which we think about things affects the way we feel, the way we behave, and our physical reactions.

Thinking negatively about living with an ostomy can make life more difficult by causing negative feelings and reactions.

There are some common themes in ostomy-related thoughts which are associated with distress and problems.

By asking yourself some questions and thinking about your negative thoughts, you can gain a new perspective on the ostomy—and this in turn can help you change your feelings and behavior.

Changing the way you think, feel, and behave about the ostomy can be difficult to do on your own; you may want to speak to your doctor or nurse about referral to a specialist, such as a clinical psychologist, for help.

Chapter 6

Coping with Your Feelings

Research has shown that approximately one-quarter of all people who have ostomy operations experience serious problems with anxiety, depression, and other negative emotions at some point during the year after their ostomy operation. Some people who have had an ostomy operation do not suffer serious problems, but may still find that there are times when they feel anxious or sad. This chapter explains some of the common features of these negative emotional reactions and also provides information on how to develop ways of coping with such feelings. The characteristics of more serious negative emotional reactions are also outlined, as these may need to be the focus of a discussion with a nurse or doctor who can arrange for professional help to improve the way you are feeling.

Anxiety

Anxiety is a common emotional reaction following ostomy surgery. You may be experiencing some of the common signs and symptoms of anxiety. This does not necessarily mean that you have a major problem; it could be part of what is called a normal adjustment reaction to the big changes that have happened in your life.

The common signs of anxiety can be divided into four types:

* physical sensations associated with anxiety

* anxious thoughts

* moods associated with anxiety

* common behavioral reactions that occur when we feel anxious

The physical sensations experienced as symptoms of anxiety include sweating, tense muscles, a pounding heart, dizziness, shortness of breath, tight chest, dry mouth, tingling, and "jelly" legs. These sensations are usually accompanied by anxious thoughts that tend to be focused on an overestimation of danger and catastrophe. The anxious thoughts are also usually related to an underestimation of your ability to cope or to obtain any help with the difficulties. The most common moods that accompany this type of thought pattern are anxiety, fear, panic, and nervousness. When people experience these moods or have anxious thoughts, they are more likely either to avoid situations in which anxiety might occur or to leave situations when they notice any of the physical sensations associated with anxiety. If you have been experiencing any of the common signs and symptoms of anxiety, it might be helpful for you to know a bit more about anxiety and where it comes from.

Anxiety is a normal human response, designed to save our lives. Our human need to respond to stress, anxiety, and fear has evolved over many thousands of years, in order to help us deal with threatening situations. Our distant ancestors faced many dangers—for example, the risk of being attacked by a saber-toothed tiger. The human body developed a response to help us escape from such dangers—you could call it a sort of "anxiety response." The physical effects of anxiety mentioned above are important parts of this anxiety response; they are designed to help us and to save our lives.

The anxiety response is automatically switched on when we are in a dangerous or threatening situation. Nowadays, very few of us are faced with threats like saber-toothed tigers, but we may be exposed to other dangers and threats: If you are crossing the road and a car comes screeching around the corner, speeding toward you, your heart beats faster, your breathing becomes faster, you get a churning in your stomach and you feel hot and sweaty.

This anxiety response can save your life by helping you get out of the way. Your heart beats faster to pump the blood to your muscles so that you can move quickly away from the car. You breathe faster because your heart needs more oxygen to keep it beating faster. Your muscles become very tense because you need to spring into action out of the way of the car. You have a churning sensation in your stomach because some of your blood has been directed to your legs from elsewhere in your body. Your body decides that your heart and legs need more blood for the emergency and that your stomach can spare some of the blood which was there. You feel hot and sweaty because of all the extra work going on inside you; your body tries to cool down by sweating. All of these physical sensations happen for very important reasons. Seeing the speeding car switches on the anxiety response, which helps you to escape from the danger and threat and therefore keeps you from harm.

In this example there was a real danger, and it was helpful that the anxiety response was switched on. However, the anxiety response can be switched on even if we only *think* something is dangerous, threatening, or difficult to cope with. You might hear a bang in the middle of the night and think there's a burglar in your house. The anxiety response is switched on even if the noise was only your cat knocking over a plant. Your thought that it may be a burglar activates the anxiety response, so you get a pounding heart, dizziness, churning stomach, and other anxiety sensations. You might get more anxious thoughts and a desire to escape.

The anxiety response is switched on when we think about danger or not being able to cope. Thoughts about danger, catastrophe, and not being able to cope commonly accompany anxious moods like fear and panic, as well as anxious behaviors like escape and avoidance. The different components of the anxiety response —physical sensations, moods, thoughts, and reactions—are all connected. Making changes in one of these components has a domino effect on the other components. This means that if you can cope with anxious thoughts, you will notice a difference in anxious moods and physical sensations. If you can cope with anxious behavior, you will also be coping with anxious physical sensations and anxious thoughts. These main components of the anxiety response are outlined below.

Anxiety Response: The Four Components

Moods:
Anxiety, fear, panic

Thoughts:
"I can't deal with this"; "What if I never get better?"; "What if it all goes wrong?"; "I'm going to collapse"

Physical sensations:
Dry mouth, dizziness, chest pain, shortness of breath, sweating, palpitations

Behavior:
Trying to escape, avoiding threatening situations

Panic is an extreme form of anxiety. Panic attacks are characterized by a period of intense fear, anxiety, or discomfort. During a panic attack, physical sensations develop and build to a peak. These sensations usually include palpitations, sweating, trembling, shortness of breath, feelings of choking, chest pain, nausea, dizziness, feelings of unreality, tingling sensations, and hot flushes. During a panic attack there is usually a feeling of impending doom (thinking that something awful is about to happen) as well as thoughts regarding personal catastrophe, such as "I'm going to die," "I'm having a heart attack," or "I'm losing my mind." These catastrophic thoughts about the normal sensations associated with anxiety and stress make things worse—you get anxious about feeling anxious. In other words, you get a tight chest because you are uptight. You then think that the tight chest means you are having a heart attack—and this makes you feel even more anxious, which makes your chest tighten up even more. You also experience even more physical sensations, such as shortness of breath and dizziness, and become convinced that your theory that you are having a heart attack is correct. This culminates in a panic attack (see Figure 3). Panic attacks are triggered by normal physical sensations

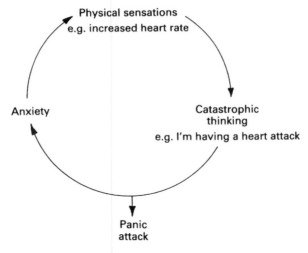

Figure 3. The vicious cycle in a panic attack

associated with being anxious. They can also be triggered by normal sensations associated with being tired or feeling unwell.

Coping with Anxiety

An effective way to cope with anxiety is to learn how to identify, evaluate, and then change the anxious thoughts that are part of the anxiety response. This way of coping with anxiety is outlined at the end of this chapter (pages 77–85), when we look at how to identify, evaluate, and change problem thoughts that are causing negative moods like anxiety and panic.

In addition to developing new ways of thinking, you can learn how to change the physical reactions of the anxiety response through relaxation techniques and breathing retraining, outlined below. Research suggests that to bring about lasting changes in anxiety problems there must be real and fundamental changes in thinking patterns. However, relaxation and breathing techniques may be helpful in the short term.

Progressive Muscle Relaxation

A common relaxation technique, called progressive muscle relaxation, involves learning to relax all the major muscle groups in your body. This combats the anxiety response by deliberately offsetting the muscle tension that is a common physical sensation of anxiety. The technique consists of tensing and then relaxing your muscles. To practice, clench one of your fists and hold it for about five seconds (don't clench too tightly—you don't want the tension to become painful). Then stop clenching and deliberately let all the tension go; relax your hand. Now pay special attention to the difference between the tension and the relaxation. Notice the warm feelings in your fist. Some people find it relaxing to say a soothing word or phrase to themselves as they release the tension from their muscles—a word or phrase such as "relax," "let go," or "release."

When you have done this a couple of times with your fist, you are ready to start on your body's main muscle groups. Get in a comfortable position, if possible either sitting or lying (you can do this technique almost anywhere). One at a time, tense and relax your biceps, feet, thighs, chest, back, shoulders, and head/face. Remember, the aim is to help you become aware of the difference between physical tension and relaxation.

Relaxation training is like learning any new skill—you won't be an expert when you begin. It will take a couple of weeks of regular practice to get used to it. You will notice that it starts to work when you set aside time to do the relaxation exercises each day. Try not to do the relaxation exercises when you are sleepy, as you may fall asleep. Start to notice in your everyday life when you are physically tense (especially around your shoulders and neck muscles). You can use this as your cue to release the tension from your muscles with the progressive relaxation technique.

Another extremely effective way of relaxing is to make a list of activities that you find (or used to find) really relaxing—such as enjoying a bubble bath, listening to a favorite piece of music, or sitting stroking the cat. Make sure you do at least three of these each day—or alternatively, to combat the anxiety response, you can do one of these activities when you are feeling particularly tense or anxious.

Breathing Retraining

When the anxiety response is switched on, we tend to breathe quickly and shallowly, which upsets the balance of oxygen and carbon dioxide in the blood. This is one of the main reasons why people get dizzy and experience a funny tingling sensation in their fingertips (paresthesia).

It is easy to bring your breathing back into balance by avoiding taking large gasps of air. First, notice whether your breathing is unbalanced. If it is, breathe in for a slow count of four, and then breathe out for a slow count of four. Repeat this three or four times. Just as unbalanced breathing was a habit, you can make balanced breathing a habit by practicing this technique.

Distraction Techniques

In the section about medical tests, we discussed the benefits of distraction in keeping your mind occupied and focused away from worrisome thoughts. You can also use distraction to cope with the physical reactions of the anxiety response. Distraction techniques are helpful for coping with anxiety responses because they focus your mind away from the thoughts that maintain anxious moods, behaviors, and physical reactions. Review the section in Chapter 3 titled "General Information" for some distraction techniques.

Antianxiety Drugs

Sometimes doctors prescribe pills to help people cope with an anxiety response. Some common antianxiety drugs are diazepam, propranolol, and buspirone. Most antianxiety drugs are prescribed only as a short-term measure, because research has shown that some of them can become addictive. We also know that when people take certain antianxiety drugs for a long time, eventually they need to take more and more to get the same effect. Drugs only take away the physical sensations—and the anxious thoughts and behavior usually return when the drugs are stopped. This is not always the case, and you should discuss your individual situation with a doctor. Antianxiety drugs may be a useful first-aid measure for anxiety symptoms, but they are not a long-term answer to anxiety for most people.

Serious Anxiety

If you are feeling anxious and/or having physical anxiety symptoms and anxious thoughts most days, or if any of these symptoms are especially unpleasant and uncontrollable, you may be suffering from an anxiety disorder that could benefit from a specialist's help. Mention this to your nurse or doctor. You should also mention if you have had panic attacks and feel worried that you will have another one. It is especially important to get help from a specialist if you notice that you are avoiding situations or have developed special rituals to protect yourself from experiencing anxiety symptoms. Effective treatments are available for most anxiety disorders.

Depression

As we saw above, the anxiety response has four components: thoughts, behavior, physical sensations, and moods. Depression—a reaction sometimes experienced following ostomy surgery—can be similarly described. The most obvious mood experienced by someone with depression is sadness—though irritability, guilt, and despair can also be problem moods in depression.

Depressed people tend to have negative thoughts about themselves (such as "I am a failure"; "I am useless"; "I am unattractive"), about the world (such as "Other people do not like me"), and about the future (such as "Things will never get any better"). When people are depressed, their behavior changes. They stop doing things they used to enjoy, they feel tired most of the time, they have problems with sleep, and they may cry a lot.

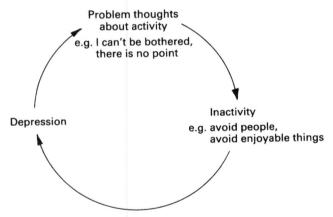

Figure 4. The vicious cycle in depression

Simple and effective strategies exist that can be used to combat the behavioral patterns that are a part of feeling depressed. However, if a person experiences serious depression, then specialized care, perhaps including treatment with anitdepressant drugs, may be called for.

Planning Activities

When people are troubled by depression they gradually become less active in general and often stop doing the activities they used to enjoy. This reduced activity level can be caused by problem thoughts such as "There's no point," "I can't be bothered," or "I won't enjoy it." Because of this negative thought pattern, depressed people grow even more inactive and thus even more depressed. This can become a vicious cycle that maintains the depressed mood, actions, and thought patterns (see Figure 4).

One way of dealing with this problem and breaking the cycle is to gradually increase the number of pleasurable activities you do in a day. Start by doing one pleasurable activity each day and build up until you are doing approximately ten pleasurable activities each week. It can be helpful to start by thinking of all the things you used to enjoy doing and making a list of them. Then pick from the list which activity you will try first. You don't need to select a time-consuming or expensive activity—anything enjoyable will do. You may be tempted to compare your pleasure with what it used to be like for you—but try not to do this. Focus on the pleasure you're getting now and how this is better than sitting around doing nothing or avoiding opportunities for enjoyment.

You will find that if you can break this vicious cycle then your mood will gradually lift. You might also find that many of the problem thoughts about not enjoying things or about there being no point in doing anything were untrue in the first place.

Serious Depression

As you read this book, you may be worried that depression is more than a passing feeling or that it is a big problem for you. You may be experiencing some of the signs and symptoms of what is called a major depressive episode, or clinical depression. If this is true, many effective treatments exist from which you can benefit, such as antidepressant drugs and cognitive therapy.

How many of the following symptoms have you experienced in the past two weeks?

* feeling depressed all day every day and being unable to "snap out of it"

* not enjoying or getting pleasure from anything you do

* problems with sleeping (an inability to fall asleep or waking up very early)

* difficulty concentrating or making decisions

* thinking about death or about killing yourself

* feeling guilty or worthless

* having a poor appetite or not enjoying food as much as you used to

If you have experienced four or more of the above signs or symptoms in the past two weeks, then you may be experiencing a clinically significant problem with depression. For a more detailed assessment, you should discuss the matter with your family physician as soon as possible.

Antidepressant Drugs

Antidepressant drugs are not addictive. They must be taken for about three weeks before they are effective, and to decrease the chances that the depression will return, they usually need to be taken for six months once the patient starts to feel better. Common examples of antidepressants include fluoxetine, amitriptyline, dothiepin, citalopram, sertraline, paroxetine, lofepramine, and trazodone—all of which are often known by their trade names.

Suicidal Thoughts

Sometimes people who are suffering from depression feel that life is not worth living or that they would be better off dead. If you have been having such thoughts, it is important that you speak to your doctor or nurse about it. Suicidal thoughts can be a symptom of depression and can be treated. People usually start thinking about suicide when they cannot think of any other way to solve their problems or because they think there are more advantages to being dead. These thoughts are always the result of distorted or biased thought processes. If you have been thinking that life is not worth living, it can be helpful to remind yourself of reasons for living. Recall a time in your life when you thought that life *was* worth living—what were your reasons for living at that time? Try to remember that these suicidal thoughts are symptoms of an illness that can be helped by treatment if you speak to your doctor.

Dealing with Feelings by Changing Your Thoughts

As we saw in the last chapter, identifying the way we think about things is very important in understanding why we have particular feelings, why we engage in certain behaviors, and why we experience certain physical reactions. Because of this link among thoughts, emotions, behavior, and physical reactions, we can produce dramatic changes by modifying the way we think about things—that is, we can alter our unhelpful feelings, actions, and physical reactions associated with anxiety or depression.

These are the basic principles behind a psychological treatment called cognitive therapy. Cognitive therapy is a "talking treatment" that aims to help the patient understand how their thinking patterns may be affecting their feelings and behavior. The patient and the cognitive therapist work together to make sense of the problematic feelings and actions, and then work on changing problematic thought patterns. Cognitive therapy has been shown to be effective in helping people who suffer from anxiety disorders or clinical depression.

The rest of this chapter outlines a method to help you identify, evaluate, and change the problem thoughts that create and feed negative and unhelpful moods, actions, and physical reactions.

There are two main steps in helping yourself deal with problem thought patterns:

1. identifying which thoughts are causing you problems

2. evaluating and changing the way in which you think about certain events or situations

Identifying and Changing Problem Thoughts

Before you can identify a problem thought, you need to identify the mood that accompanies it and that you would like to change. This poses no problems for some people. However, others find it difficult to know what feeling or emotion they are experiencing, and how to describe it. It can be helpful to spend a few days "tuning in" to your emotions. You can do this by making a mental note of what emotion you are experiencing at different points during the day. Ask yourself, "What am I feeling right now?" You may find it helpful to look at the emotion checklist below as you start to become aware of and tune in to your emotions.

Emotion Checklist

This is a checklist of negative emotions. Look at the list to see if you can identify any emotions that bother you and that you might want to alter by changing your thinking patterns:

* worry

* anxiety

* depression

* anger

* frustration

* fear

* panic

* irritability

* shame

* guilt

* sadness

After you have spent some time tuning in to your emotions, you will notice that you experience many different moods—some positive, some negative; some that involve strong emotions, and others that have less of a grip on you. It is probably the strong negative emotions that you want to learn to cope with. Throughout this book, I have recommended writing things down. Writing down information about your feelings and thoughts can be a helpful tool in remembering the details of how you were feeling or what you were thinking about.

If you notice a negative mood (e.g., depression), think about how strong the mood is. Give it a score from zero to 100 percent. A score of zero would mean not depressed at all, while a score of 100 percent would mean the most depressed you could ever imagine feeling. Can you think of a strong negative mood that you have had recently? Score its strength using a scale of zero to 100 percent. Scoring the negative mood is an important part of identifying and changing your problem thoughts, so that you can rate your moods before and after your attempt to change your problem thoughts and thereby gauge the improvement.

Once you start to notice negative moods that you want to change, you are ready to start looking for problem thoughts. Negative moods are always accompanied by problem thoughts. When you notice that you are having a strong negative mood (e.g., depressed: 85 percent), write it down—along with its score—on a Problem-Thought Record (an example and some blank forms appear toward the end of this chapter). Write a brief description of the situation you are in when the negative mood happens: Where are you? Who else is present? What are you doing or saying?

You can now start to find the problem thought that is behind the negative mood. The best way to find problem thoughts is to ask yourself some simple—but tried and tested—questions. Remember, it is problem thoughts that make problem moods stay with you. If you can learn to identify the problem thoughts, then you are well on the way to coping with the problem moods.

Questions for Identifying Problem Thoughts

Whenever you experience a problem mood, ask yourself the following questions to help you identify the problem thoughts behind the mood:

1. What was going through my mind just as I started to have this problem mood?

2. What does this situation mean to me? What does this situation say about me?

3. What is the worst thing that could happen in this situation?

4. What have I just been thinking about?

5. What do I guess that I was thinking about just then?

Write down the answers to these questions on your Problem-Thought Record, under the heading "Problem thought(s)." These answers will contain the problem thoughts that are feeding the problem mood.

When you have identified a list of problem thoughts, you can work to modify them to create a more helpful way of thinking about things. It has been shown that when patients use this technique regularly, strong moods become less intense (e.g., "depressed: 85 percent" becomes "depressed: 25 percent"), and they experience the negative moods less often. Because moods are linked to actions and physical reactions, there is a domino effect: Changing thoughts changes moods, which change actions and physical reactions. In order to modify the problem thoughts, you need to "try on" a different perspective. To do this, you can learn to ask yourself some different questions, designed to change the problem thoughts (these are provided in "Questions for Changing Problem Thoughts," below).

Common Thinking Biases

Problem thoughts are often the result of biases or distortions in thinking. These biases or distortions have special names. When you begin to change problem thoughts, it can be helpful to look for these biases. Some common biases are described below.

All-or-nothing thinking: seeing things in black-and-white categories—either everything is going completely well or it is a complete disaster. There are no shades of gray when this type of thinking bias is operating. An example of all-or-nothing thinking would be, "These ostomy bags are completely useless."

Overgeneralization: seeing a single event as part of a never-ending pattern of events, or generalizing from one isolated event to the rest of our lives. Thoughts such as, "My bag always leaks when I go out," when you have experienced one or two leaks, or, "Everything is going wrong with my ostomy," when you get an area of sore skin—these are examples of thoughts that are a result of overgeneralization.

Mental filter: picking out a single negative detail and focusing on it exclusively. An example of this would be focusing on, "The surgeon said I might develop some problems later on"—and forgetting that he also said that this was unlikely and that there were many effective treatments if problems did develop.

Discounting the positive: believing that positive experiences don't count. If you feel your energy level increasing after surgery, you might say to yourself, "So what? I am still apprehensive about going out and meeting people." This is an example of discounting the positive.

Jumping to conclusions: drawing conclusions when there are no facts to support the conclusion. *Mind reading* is an example of this—you make predictions about what other people think as if you had mind-reading abilities. Thoughts such as "They are not interested in visiting me" or "They think I smell" are examples of this. *Fortune-telling* is another bias that involves jumping to conclusions. This involves predicting that something won't work out—"I'll never get used to this stoma" or, "swimming will never be the same again" are examples of the fortune-telling bias. You think these thoughts as if you can really see into the future.

Magnification: exaggerating the importance of your difficulties and problems and minimizing your abilities to cope and your positive qualities. A thought like, "Being more confident about the appliance is no big deal—I still feel awkward wearing it" is a result of the magnification bias.

Emotional reasoning: assuming that our negative feelings are a reflection of the way things really are. You may be saying to yourself, "I feel that everyone is looking at me" or "I feel that people can see my ostomy through my clothes." This bias causes us to confuse feelings with facts. Because you *feel* a certain way, you believe reality *is* that way.

Personalization: holding yourself personally responsible for an event that is not entirely under your control. You may think, "The doctor spoke to me for only a few minutes because I was not explaining things clearly," when the doctor might simply have been busier than usual.

Questions for Changing Problem Thoughts

Once you have identified the situation, the problem mood, and the problem thoughts and have written them down on your Problem-Thought Record, you can start working to change the thoughts as a way of improving how you feel. Just as you can identify problem thoughts by asking yourself a set of questions, so you can also modify your problem thoughts by asking yourself a series of questions. Ask yourself the questions listed below. Write your answers on the Problem-Thought Record, under the heading "More helpful, alternative thoughts."

1. What experiences have I had which show me that this thought is not completely true all of the time?

2. If I were trying to help someone I cared about to feel better when they had this thought, what would I say to them?

3. What advice might someone I cared about give me if they knew I was thinking about things in this way? Would they agree with me? If not, why not?

4. When I am not experiencing this problem mood, how do I think about things?

5. What have I learned from previous events or experiences that might help me to cope with this problem thought?

6. Is my problem thought an example of a thinking bias? If so, which one?

7. What is the evidence to support this thought? What is the evidence against this thought?

8. What is the worst thing that could happen? Could I live through and cope with this?

9. What is the best thing that could happen? What is the most realistic outcome?

10. What would be the effect of changing this problem thought? What can I do now?

Problem-Thought Record

You should now have a better idea about how to identify and modify problem thoughts and moods. Below is an example of a completed Problem-Thought Record followed by a blank Problem-Thought Record for you to complete. If you want to know more about these techniques, get a copy of *Mind over Mood* (see "Further Reading" in "Resources," at the end of the book).

Problem-Thought Record (Example)

Day/date/situation: Monday, March 25
   Sitting watching TV program about surgical operations

Problem mood(s):
   depressed: 65 percent

   frustrated: 50 percent

Problem thought(s):
   [This is where you write your answers from "Questions for Identifying Problem Thoughts," above.]

   I can't be bothered getting dressed.

   I will never get over this operation and be normal again.

   I have no energy to visit Mark today—I won't enjoy it anyway.

More helpful, alternative thoughts:
   [This is where you write your answers from "Questions for Changing Problem Thoughts," above.]

   If someone I knew thought this, I would advise them to get dressed—they would feel better once they did it.

   I am predicting the future in a negative way, and this isn't going to help.

   When I don't feel this way, I tell myself I just need to take it easy and one step at a time—be kind to myself.

   My thoughts are affected by biases like fortune-telling and emotional reasoning—I can try to reverse these biases.

   If I try, then I might find some energy. I don't know for sure that I won't enjoy it until I try.

Problem mood(s) now:
   depressed: 20 percent

   frustrated: 10 percent

Problem-Thought Record

Day/date/situation:

....

....

Problem mood(s):

....

....

....

Problem thought(s):

....

....

....

....

More helpful, alternative thoughts:

....

....

....

....

....

....

Problem mood(s) now:

....

....

Make copies of this format for additional records

Summary

Anxiety is a common reaction following an ostomy operation and can be understood by looking at its four components: physical sensations, moods, thoughts, and actions. Anxiety is characterized by physical sensations such as dizziness and dry mouth, moods such as fear and panic, thoughts such as "I can't cope with this" and "I'm going to collapse," and actions such as avoidance and escape.

The human anxiety response developed to save us from danger, but it can also be switched on when we simply *think* that a situation is dangerous, even if it isn't.

Anxiety responses can be dealt with using strategies such as breathing retraining and progressive muscle relaxation; antianxiety drugs may also be used as a short-term measure.

Depression can also be understood in terms of four components: physical sensations such as loss of appetite, moods such as sadness and irritability, thoughts such as "I'm a failure" and "Life is a mess," and actions such as withdrawing from others and becoming inactive.

Depression can be helped by gradually increasing activity levels and planning enjoyable activities that give a sense of achievement. Antidepressant medication may also be helpful for some people.

Clinical depression is more serious and requires consultation with your physician.

Problem thoughts are one of the main causes of negative moods after ostomy surgery. You can learn some simple techniques for identifying emotions and problem thoughts and for modifying the problem thoughts to help you feel better.

Chapter 7

Dealing with Social Situations

Some of the most common concerns of people with an ostomy have to do with social and public situations. You may worry that the bag will come off or leak when you're in a public situation, that the ostomy will make embarrassing noises when you least expect it, that it will give off an unpleasant smell, or that other people will notice the bag underneath your clothing. Some of these thoughts have already been mentioned, but this chapter provides specific advice about worries regarding social situations and outlines several techniques for dealing with such concerns.

Worries about the ostomy being detected, and about other people thinking negatively of you, can make it difficult to get used to being in social situations after your operation. Moira had an ileostomy and was afraid that her ostomy would give off a foul smell or make an unexpected noise if she went to visit Mike. She thought she couldn't possibly cope with this. She also believed that Mike would think she was dirty and rude if he noticed the smell or heard the noise. Because of these thoughts, she felt anxious, dizzy, and tense and her heart was racing. She decided to avoid visiting Mike.

Moira's worries about this social situation are maintained by her thoughts that she'll have a problem if she visits Mike, that she won't be able to cope with the problem if it occurs, and that Mike will think less of her because of the problem. It is not surprising that she doesn't go to visit Mike and that she feels anxiety sensations as a result of these problem thoughts. Yet Moira could modify these thoughts by using a Problem-Thought Record. This would likely be helpful, as there are a number of thinking biases in her thoughts about this social situation. What biases can you spot in Moira's thought processes?

In addition to identifying and modifying the thoughts that underlie the desire to avoid social situations and the worries about such situations, other techniques exist to help you cope with these issues. It is all too easy to focus on the worst possible scenario and to underestimate what you could do to cope if the worst were to happen. How does this work? You keep thinking that the worst will happen (though you may be overestimating the chances that it will)—and your thinking stops there. You don't think further about whether you could realistically do anything to cope if it actually *did* happen.

What Is the Worst Thing That Can Happen?

Social anxiety usually occurs when you believe that something will go wrong in a social situation. You may worry that your ostomy will make a noise or that you will smell. You may imagine that your bag will leak all over your clothes in the middle of the supermarket or that noises might erupt from the bag during prayers at church. It is natural to have these sorts of worries after an ostomy operation. However, such worries can become a problem if you start to feel really apprehensive and to avoid doing things you enjoy. This can be one of the first signs of clinical depression.

Think for a moment about what the worst thing is that could happen to you. Try to think about it in great detail. What would happen? How would you feel? What would your ostomy be doing? What would you say? How would other people react?

Now that you have an idea about the worst-case scenario, ask yourself if this is likely to happen. Might you be overestimating how likely it is? How many times have you been in similar situations and been okay?

"I Couldn't Cope If That Happened"

Now that you have thought about the worst-case scenario, you will probably realize that you have been overestimating the likelihood of the worst happening. This exercise might also have triggered thoughts and worries that you could not possibly cope if the worst were indeed to occur. Accidents and unplanned incidents do happen. Instead of assuming that you couldn't cope, why not make a coping plan now, before it happens? Instead of stopping your thought process after you have considered the worst possibility, take it forward and construct a coping plan.

Write down your worst-case scenario for a social situation on the left side of a piece of paper, and then on the right side of the same piece of paper write down what you could do to cope if it were to happen. This might be difficult, but you can make it easier by thinking about what other people might do to cope—or by asking some people you trust about what they might do. This exercise helps you to see that there are things you could do to cope if your fears were to come true. Not only that, but you are also thinking about a coping plan in advance so that if something awful were to happen, you would be prepared in advance. You wouldn't have to think on the spot—you would have worked it all out beforehand. In other words, you just put the coping plan into action as you have prepared it. This technique can also be used for worst-case scenarios in other areas of life—such as future illness, family problems, or visiting friends. I know some couples who devise a special code word to indicate to each other that an accident has occurred.

Some examples of worst-case scenarios with coping plans are outlined below.

Worst-Case Scenarios and Coping Plans

The bag will come off and the contents start to run down my leg.

* I can excuse myself and go to the bathroom to clean myself up. I can then go home and change.

Norma will ask me about my ostomy when I don't want to talk about it.

* I can say that I appreciate her concerns but that I am not ready to talk about it to other people yet.

The ostomy will make loud noises when everyone is quiet, and I will feel so embarrassed.

* I could say, "Oh—excuse me," or I could say when I arrive that my operation causes my bowel to sometimes make noises. I can remind myself that people have previously been really understanding.

The ostomy will balloon with air and there will be a bulge under my dress. There might be a smell.

* I can go to the bathroom and let the air out. I can remind myself that it is unlikely that anyone else will have noticed.

Remember, even if your worst fears do come true, there is always something you can do to cope. Most likely you will never have to use your coping plan, but at least you know it is there if you need it. Most people say they find it easier to put into action a plan they've already thought about, rather than having to improvise when something happens.

Use the spaces below to write down your worst-case scenarios and your coping plans.

Worst-Case Scenario

....

....

Coping Plan

....

....

Worst-Case Scenario

....

....

Coping Plan

....

....

Worst-Case Scenario

....

....

Coping Plan

....

....

"I Don't Know What to Tell Other People"

Some of my patients have dealt with worries over telling other people about their ostomy by practicing what to say to them. In this way, they can think of *how* to say it and thereby take control of the social situation. Some, for example, find it helpful to explain about their ostomy as soon as they enter a new social situation. One man told me this was his way of making sure other people knew what was happening if there was an embarrassing noise. This might seem difficult, but once you have thought out what you want to say to someone, you can practice it beforehand. Many people prefer not to say anything—but even so, this strategy of planning and practicing what to say may be the key to reducing your worries about what others will think.

Here is an example of how one patient handled it:

> As you know, I have been very ill. To save my life I had a colostomy operation—that means I have to wear a bag on my tummy. It sometimes makes some funny noises— which can be a bit embarrassing. I hope you don't mind my telling you this, but I feel less anxious if I explain this in advance.

He found that most people were extremely understanding when he said this.

It is unlikely that other people will notice either the bag or any smell it gives off (other people's noses are much further away from it than yours is). Osotmy patients who have come to my clinic with social anxiety seem to think that their friends and acquaintances are not going to be understanding. However, they then tell me that they themselves would understand if someone they knew had an ostomy. If you have explained to someone about your operation, how could they possibly fail to be understanding of the fact that you have experienced major, life-saving surgery?

Action, Not Avoidance

You might be scared about going on long trips to see friends or about staying for a while at someone's house. This is probably because you have lost some control over your bowel or bladder. One way to overcome this is with a gradual approach, whereby you work gently toward getting back to the way you were before the operation. In other words, you don't have to jump in at the deep end; your first outing after the operation doesn't have to be a big social occasion, like a high school reunion or the golf club dinner-dance—instead, you can work up to these sorts of events slowly. This is a very important technique for dealing with anxiety-provoking situations; it is called graded exposure.

Here is an example of the graded-exposure steps made by one ostomy patient who was feeling anxious about going out because of her appliance:

Final goal: Go to Sheila's coffee gathering on June 13

Step #	Description	Date(s)	Anxiety rating (0–10) predicted	actual
1.	Go into the corner shop	4 June	6	4
		5 June	5	3
2.	Visit Doreen	6 June	8	4
3.	Go to the post office	8 June	7	3
		9 June	5	3
4.	Go to the supermarket	9 June	4	2
		10 June	4	2
5.	Go to Sheila's coffee gathering	13 June	5	1

This woman thought about what she wanted to be able to do (go to the coffee gathering on 13 June) and then devised a plan to help her work toward her goal gradually. If you think this technique might be helpful, first of all think about what activity you would like to be able to do. Then break it down into smaller steps. Now you are ready to start a gradual approach to reaching your goal. Note: The key is to keep repeating a step until you feel comfortable enough to move on to the next step.

By keeping a note of how anxious she thought she would be and how anxious she actually was, this woman could also see that she was overestimating her anxiety levels. She was fortune-telling, in terms of her thinking bias. Every time you take a step, keep a note of how anxious you thought beforehand you would be, and then how anxious you actually were.

Remember to keep repeating each step until you are ready for the next one. If you move on too quickly, don't worry—just go back to the previous step until you feel ready to move on. You might also want to think of a more gradual step forward, in case your previous step was too ambitious.

Below is a space to write in your own graded-exposure steps for working toward a social goal.

Final goal:

....

....

Step #   Description   Date(s)   Anxiety rating (0–10)
                                                       predicted   actual

1. ....

....

2. ....

....

3. ....

....

4. ....

....

5. ....

....

Becoming Less Self-Conscious

You might notice that, since the operation, you have become acutely self-conscious, with your attention completely focused on your ostomy and how you are feeling physically. This means you are more aware of it and thus more prone to start thinking that the ostomy will make a noise and/or smell. You can cope with this self-conscious tendency by deliberately directing your attention to what is going on around you. This helps, because you become less aware of the ostomy and what it is up to. One way of directing your attention away from your bodily sensations is to focus on what other people are wearing, what they are saying, whether you like their clothes, hairstyles, etc.

Your anxiety about social situations may be so overpowering that you find it difficult to overcome. It may interfere with your usual routine—your return to work and/or your social life. Indeed, it may be so bad that you stay at home all the time or that you have a panic attack in social situations. If this sounds like you, discuss the matter with your ET or physician. They may recommend that you see a clinical psychologist about this more serious form of social anxiety.

Summary

Worries about ostomy smells or noises can make social situations difficult to cope with.

Recording your thoughts in social situations, and then developing alternative ways of thinking, can help you to feel less anxious in social situations. Use the Problem-Thought Record from Chapter 6 to guide you through this process.

Thinking in advance about possible problems (the worst-case scenario) and how to cope with them is an excellent way of dealing with your worst fears.

Explaining to other people about the ostomy can make you less worried about what they might think if you have a problem with the ostomy while you're with them.

If you feel anxious about attending a social event, consider taking a gradual approach, starting with a more low-key situation and then building up to a busier one.

Switching the focus of your attention away from yourself and on to what is going on around you can be an effective way of dealing with self-consciousness (i.e., your tendency to focus on the ostomy).

Chapter 8

Sex, Intimacy, and Life with an Ostomy

My initial concerns about my ostomy related to its appearance and the worries I had about intimacy. I was very aware of the pouch, even the mini-pouch that is available. My fears were conveyed to my partner, resulting in less intimacy between us. It took longer than I expected to get used to this.

Female with ileostomy, age 40

Humans often find it difficult to talk openly about sexual matters and intimate relationships. Health-care professionals are humans, and despite the fact that they may have had some training in this area, they still may find it difficult to talk to their patients about sex and intimacy. This is unfortunate, as ostomates inevitably want to talk about intimate relationships at some point before or after the operation.

This chapter outlines some of the main issues that affect the intimate relationships of people with ostomies. First, we will look at the worries ostomy patients may have over what to say to a new partner about their ostomy. Next, we will consider the worries people may develop about the effect of the ostomy on an existing relationship. The chapter then focuses on human sexual responses, some of the problems that can develop following an ostomy operation, and strategies for overcoming problems in this area.

Sex and intimacy have different degrees of importance in people's lives. This may not be an area of major concern for you—and therefore you may not feel the need to read this chapter. Some readers may be shocked by the explicit nature of parts of this chapter, but to shock is not my intention. I make no apology for highlighting sex and intimacy as an important part of life with an ostomy. I have encountered too many patients who did not receive appropriate information on this aspect of their lives because health-care professionals could not overcome their own embarrassment. I also know of patients who were afraid to ask for details and health-care professionals who made sweeping generalizations about a particular patient's life (such as, "They won't be interested in that sort of thing at their age").

What Should I Tell a Future Partner?

If you are not in an intimate relationship before ostomy surgery, you may be very worried about how you will tell a potential partner about your ostomy. Most people in this situation find it difficult to know whether to talk about the ostomy right from the moment they meet someone to whom they are attracted or whether to wait until there is a possibility of sexual intimacy. Some people are surprised to find out that, after weeks of worrying about what to say, when to say it, and how to say it, their new partner already knows about it from a friend or relative.

Remember that most people do not even know what an ostomy is. This can be an advantage, as they will take their lead from you. If you tell them about it in a matter-of-fact way that suggests you have no problems with it, they will have nothing to be concerned about. They will see that you are not concerned—and therefore that they do not need to be either. Everyone has a different way of dealing with this potentially awkward situation.

The important thing is to think about all the options open to you and to weigh the advantages and disadvantages of each option in advance. This is called a cost-benefit analysis. If you are finding it difficult to decide what to say to a future partner, you can think of the advantages and disadvantages of some of the options listed below. Beside each option, write down what you see as its advantages and disadvantages. This will help you decide what feels best for you.

Cost-Benefit Analysis

1. Do not tell them about it at all.

Advantages:

....

....

Disadvantages:

....

....

2. If I like them, tell them immediately.

Advantages:

....

....

Disadvantages:

....

....

3. Tell them once I feel the relationship is going in that direction.

Advantages:

....

....

Disadvantages:

....

....

4. Wait until the last possible minute—when they need to know.

Advantages:

....

....

Disadvantages:

....

....

Most people decide that telling a potential partner as soon as possible is the preferred option. They reason that if they feel warmly toward someone, they would like to find out as soon as possible how their potential partner feels about the ostomy. This way they can avoid being hurt too much, because the relationship is in the early stages. However, you may wish to think of another strategy—one that may be better for you and for your particular life situation or potential partner.

You might want to think about "rehearsing" your preferred option to make it easier when the situation actually arises. You might even want to go over what you plan to say with a friend; this can be helpful because it lets you try out different ways of saying things and can boost your confidence about how to tell a potential partner.

Once you have decided on your preferred option, you can think about all of the possible responses you might receive from the other person. Then, consider how you will respond to their reactions. That way, you will be prepared for whatever happens, rather than having to think of an instant response.

For example:

Chosen option: Discuss the subject when I feel the relationship is going that way.

Possible reaction: They will say nothing about it and change the subject.

What I'll do: I can say that it is important to me to talk about how they feel about it.

Possible reaction: They say they already knew because a mutual friend told them.

What I'll do: I can ask how they feel about it.

Most people report positive experiences of telling other people about their ostomy. Common reactions are: "Is that all?" or "Why are you telling me that—I'm not bothered by it" or "I don't care about that; I love you as a person." However, it is important to remember that there is a remote possibility that the person you tell may not wish to continue with the relationship. Obviously, you hope that this will not happen. But the possibility must be mentioned, as rejection of this kind can be a severe blow—especially if you have had to deal with rejection before or if you have a negative view of yourself. If the person does not wish the relationship to continue, it might be helpful to consider whether it is better to find out at this stage instead of months later. Would you really have wanted to continue in a relationship with someone who is so bothered by the ostomy? Try not to start thinking that you must be flawed as a person and that this means you will never have a relationship again. You might want to talk the experience over with a trusted friend, if it does occur.

Will My Present Partner Reject Me?

If you were already involved in an intimate relationship before having ostomy surgery, you may have worried about its effects on your relationship—that your partner will not find you attractive following surgery or will reject you. Whatever your concerns about the effect of the ostomy on your relationship, try to talk them over with each other. You may be surprised to find that this is enough in itself to make you both feel better about the situation. You might also want to talk things over with someone whom you feel you can confide in—perhaps a friend, a relative, or one of the health professionals you know, such as your ET or doctor.

Sometimes, worries about rejection by a partner are a reflection of thoughts you have about yourself, such as, "I feel unattractive." These thoughts do not usually reflect what other people actually think of you. If you are thinking this way, you probably are employing the thinking bias of mind-reading, that is, believing your partner thinks a certain way without even discussing it with them.

It can be easy to focus on only one piece of information and blow it out of proportion. You might want to use a Problem-Thought Record (Chapter 6) to identify the problem thoughts behind the problem feelings in your relationship. You may have noticed that you have become very self-conscious, preferring to get undressed in the dark, avoiding mirrors, diving under the covers to avoid being seen, or locking the bathroom door to avoid your partner seeing you.

Some people find that their ostomy adds to relationship difficulties that were already present. In my experience, relationship breakdown following ostomy surgery is almost always due to problems that already existed in the relationship before the operation. Relationship problems may benefit from professional help, such as marriage counselling.

Sexual Aspects of Relationships

Whether or not you were involved in a relationship before the ostomy operation, you probably have some questions or concerns about intimacy and the sexual aspects of relationships. First, we will look at the basic elements of human sexual response, then at some of the sexual problems that can occur following ostomy surgery. Strategies to help with concerns regarding these issues will then be discussed.

The Human Sexual Response

Masters and Johnson, two famous researchers in the area of human sexual behavior, determined that our sexual responses can be divided into five main stages. These stages are characterized by desire, excitement, plateau, orgasm, and resolution. It is helpful to understand the main features of these stages before considering some of the problems that can follow an ostomy operation.

The *desire* stage of the human sexual response is characterized by thoughts, fantasies, and urges to engage in sexual activity. You are experiencing this stage if you are "in the mood" for sex. Sexual desire can be triggered by internal or external cues. An example of an external cue is seeing your partner naked after a shower or smelling a favorite fragrance that you associate with him or her. An example of an internal cue is thinking about cuddling your partner or recalling a pleasant event you've shared.

The next stage of the human sexual response is called the *excitement* stage. During this stage, various physical changes occur within the body that enable sexual intercourse to take place (assuming this is desired by both partners). In men, this stage is characterized by increased blood flow to the penis (the penis lengthens, becoming hard and erect) and a general increase in overall physical arousal that causes increased blood pressure, heart rate, and breathing rate. In women, the sexual excitement stage is characterized by the same general increase in overall arousal and by increased blood flow to the vagina. The vagina also lengthens.

The excitement stage is followed by the *plateau* stage, when there is a levelling off of arousal. It is during this third stage that men experience what is called ejaculatory inevitability. This means that the man knows he is going to ejaculate (or "come").

The fourth stage is *orgasm*. During this stage, women experience a sense of intense pleasure, accompanied by rhythmic contractions of the muscles around the base of the vagina. In men, rhythmic contractions of the urethra (see Chapter 1) propel semen (sperm) outwards.

The fifth and final stage of the human sexual response is called the *resolution* stage. In both men and women, this stage is characterized by a general calming down and a feeling of relaxation. In men, there is a rapid loss of erection, and for a period of time there is little response to further stimulation. Further ejaculation is impossible (the refractory period).

You probably recognize these stages from your own sexual experiences. Knowing about them makes it easier to understand any problems that develop, as you can pinpoint the stage at which the problem is happening.

Sexual Intimacy After Ostomy Surgery

Most people find that with time they forget about the ostomy during sexual intimacy. You may remember the first time you had to wear glasses or had a new hairstyle. You were initially very conscious about the change, but as time went on you noticed that you (and other people) became less aware of it. This process is called habituation. The same thing happens with your self-consciousness about the ostomy and the appliance during intimacy.

Remember that you have had major surgery and that you should resume sexual activity gradually. It is probably best to wait until your abdominal wound has healed before you engage in full sexual intercourse again. It is a good idea to ensure that the appliance is emptied before sexual intimacy and that it is securely in place. You may also want to consider wearing a smaller appliance at this time if possible. Some people roll their appliance upwards and tape it to their abdomen to keep it from getting in the way. Appliance covers can be bought to camouflage the pouch; these may help if you are concerned about this aspect.

A partner may be worried that the ostomy will be damaged during sexual intimacy. You can reassure them that this is not the case. The ostomy should never be used as part of sexual activity (for example, attempting to insert fingers or a penis into the ostomy). If you are worried about intercourse, then perhaps as a couple you can have an agreement that, to start with, you will restrict your intimate moments to hugging, kissing, and touching. This way the pressure is off, and you don't need to worry that things are going to progress too fast for you. It can be helpful to remember (especially in the early stages after surgery) that there is more to intimacy than sexual intercourse (baths, showers, massage, kissing, cuddling, etc.). Patience, communication, and mutual understanding are the key components to overcoming concerns about sexual intimacy following surgery. Expect some awkward moments and a few setbacks. Try to see these as opportunities for you to grow closer as a couple.

All the information in this chapter applies equally to heterosexual and homosexual intimacy. The issues and facts relating to lesbian sex and gay male sex are exactly the same—the ostomy need not be an obstacle to a satisfying and mutually fulfilling sexual relationship. Some people who have had an ostomy operation may have undergone an abdominoperineal resection (see Chapter 1), in which their rectum and anal passage are closed. For a man who has previously enjoyed anal intercourse with a partner, this may be a difficult part of adjusting to life with an ostomy. However, most men who have sex with men can enjoy pleasurable and fulfilling sexual relationships by other means after stoma surgery, such as oral sex and mutual masturbation. (There is a tendency for heterosexuals to assume that men who have sex with men only ever engage in anal intercourse. This illustrates a common problem in understanding sexual intimacy: Never make assumptions.)

Sexual Problems After Ostomy Surgery

Ostomy surgery can involve the risk of damaging nerves in the body that are involved in sexual functioning. If you have not been given information about whether this applies to you, contact your ET or your surgeon for more details. It may be that your particular operation does not involve damage to these important nerves. But if there is a possibility of such damage occurring, you may have to adjust to changes in the sexual aspects of your relationships. I would emphasize the word *changes*. Physical damage to important nerves does not mean the sexual aspects of your relationship have disappeared. It might mean that you and your partner need to develop new ways of enjoying sexual intimacy.

Problems with sexual functioning can be caused by factors other than nerve damage. Feelings, thoughts, alcohol, and some medications can have negative effects on sexual functioning. If you recognize any of the problems discussed below, a detailed assessment by a suitably qualified professional will identify which aspects are important for you. Discuss this with your ET or your physician.

Some of the sexual problems that can follow ostomy surgery can be helped when they are identified—especially if you think of these problems in terms of the stages of the human sexual response outlined above.

Reduced Sex Drive

Some people who have had ostomy operations notice that they lose their interest in sexual activity, that they have no desire for sex anymore. Remember that you are advised to take it easy and resume sexual activities gradually—your interest may take a few weeks to return. However, if your desire for sexual activity has not returned two months after you leave the hospital, you might consider speaking to your doctor about it.

A reduced sexual desire can affect both men and women, and it is generally associated with other changes in the relationship. A more extreme version of this problem involves a strong aversion to any sexual contact.

Problems can also develop with sexual arousal, whereby men may have difficulties gaining an erection and women may experience a lack of excitement and vaginal lubrication.

Difficulty with Erections

Men may notice that they have difficulty in getting an erection or in keeping it until the completion of sexual activity. This problem is usually accompanied by a lack of sexual excitement or pleasure. You may have heard people refer to this problem as *impotence* (or *erectile dysfunction*). Impotence is particularly common among men who have had a cystectomy operation (removal of the urinary bladder) with a urostomy. These problems with erections can occur following an ostomy operation if the surgery has damaged the nerves that control erection. However, a man who has problems with erections does not necessarily have problems with ejaculation. This is because ejaculation and erection are controlled by different nerves within the body.

Difficulty with Orgasm

Achieving orgasm may be difficult for a man or a woman, and men may also experience problems with premature ejaculation. This means that the man will ejaculate before he wants to, or in response to very little stimulation.

Painful Intercourse

Sexual intercourse can become associated with pain (called *dyspareunia*). This problem is more common in women, although it can occur in men. The pain usually occurs when the man inserts his penis into the vagina, or during thrusting. The pain is typically experienced near the opening of the vagina or deep inside the vagina. This sort of pain after an ostomy operation is almost always due to scar tissue that has developed after surgery. It can be very distressing for the person experiencing it, and the pain can occur before, during, or after intercourse. Some women develop a disorder called *vaginismus*—this involves recurrent or persistent spasms of the muscles on the outside of the vagina, which interfere with sexual intercourse.

General Treatments

All of the above problems can be very distressing to the person experiencing them and to their sexual partner, especially if they had a fulfilling sexual relationship before the surgery. The good news is there are effective treatments for most of these problems, and if you tell your doctor or nurse about the problem, they can refer you to a specialist for assessment and treatment. If you are troubled or worried by any of the above, you should have a further assessment. However, there may be some things you can do in the meantime to try to help with the problem. We shall now look at some simple strategies for dealing with sexual intimacy problems, such as impotence, vaginismus, and pain.

The key to preventing major difficulties in any relationship is honest and open communication. Communication is an essential part of intimate relationships—you need to be able to tell your partner about your worries, how you feel, what you enjoy, etc. This may be particularly important as you both take it easy after surgery—you can tell him/her what is comfortable, what you find stimulating, what you would like him/her to do more of, etc.

Pain associated with sexual intercourse can often be helped by adopting different sexual positions. Problems with erections can also be helped if partners change sexual positions—for example, a man who has erectile problems could try having intercourse lying on his back, with his female partner sitting astride him. There are other ways in which erections can be achieved, some of which are outlined below. Speak to your doctor if you think you or your partner could benefit from some advice.

Prescription Medications

Sildenafil (Viagra) increases the body's ability to achieve and maintain an erection during sexual stimulation and is prescribed for and successful in the vast majority of cases.

Glyceryl Trinitrate Patches

These patches are stuck onto the skin of the penis. They enlarge the blood vessels, allowing more blood to flow through the penis so that it becomes erect.

Vacuum Devices

Vacuum devices consist of a cylinder which is placed over the penis; a pump then extracts air from the cylinder. This produces a partial vacuum, which draws blood into the penis and produces an erection. A rubber ring is then rolled from the cylinder onto the base of the penis. The rings stops blood from leaving the penis, thus allowing the erection to be maintained. Because the ring is in place, the cylinder can be taken off. It is also possible to obtain a condom vacuum device that does the same job and is worn during sexual intercourse.

Injections

The blood flow to the penis can be increased by injecting drugs directly into the penis. Injections need to be repeated whenever an erection is required.

Implant Operations

Plastic rods may be surgically inserted into the penis. These rods can be semirigid, to give a permanent erection, or flexible so that they can be moved when necessary. It is also possible to obtain an inflatable device whereby cylinders are implanted in the penis and a pump mechanism is implanted in the scrotal sac. Implant surgery of this type can be complicated by problems such as infection or rejection.

If you are interested in finding out about these various ways of helping with erectile problems, speak to your family doctor, who can either help you directly or refer you to a specialist in psycho-sexual medicine.

Lubrication

If a woman experiences problems producing or maintaining an adequate amount of lubrication within the vagina, a lubricant such as KY Jelly or Astroglide usually leads to a significant improvement. (If you and your partner use condoms as a contraception or to protect against sexually transmitted diseases, make sure you use a lubricant that will not damage the condom.) Some of my female patients have solved this problem by using their own or their partner's saliva. This solution may not appeal to you. Remember that, as with most aspects of sexual relationships and especially intimacy after ostomy surgery, almost anything goes so long as you and your partner feel comfortable with it.

"I Could Never Speak to My Doctor About Sex"

After reading this chapter, you may have decided that it would be helpful to speak to your doctor or nurse about a sexual problem or another aspect of an intimate relationship. But you might be worried about this—and the worry may act as a barrier preventing you from taking the first step. Most of us at some point have been embarrassed when needing to talk about our sexual behavior to someone else. When I see patients with sexual problems, I always explain that I understand that they might feel embarrassed or uncomfortable at first, but that I have talked with many people about intimate problems and that their embarrassment will decrease with time. Tell your doctor if you are concerned about intimacy; he or she can assess the problem, and you will soon feel at ease discussing the best ways to help.

Graded Reintroduction of Sexual Intimacy

The general treatment advice given above may not be enough to enable you and your partner to overcome worries and concerns about the sexual aspects of your relationship. You might want to consider trying a gradual self-help program to help you build intimacy back into your relationship. This book has emphasized that so much of living with an ostomy involves taking things one step at a time. A gradual approach to sexual intimacy is crucial, as you may find that you have sexual urges before sexual responses have returned.

One of the main causes of problems with sexual intimacy and functioning is performance anxiety. This can be particularly difficult for those who have had an ostomy operation. Not only are they anxious about how *they* will perform, but they are also concerned about how the ostomy, the ostomy appliance, and their partner will "perform." Problems with sexual desire, sexual arousal, and performance anxiety can be tackled by gradually increasing sexual intimacy.

A graded approach is especially helpful in enabling people who have had ostomy surgery to regain their levels of enjoyment of sexual intimacy. To start with, you and your partner should agree that sexual intercourse is not your first aim. Your first aim is to use gentle and sensual touching as a way of beginning to feel comfortable with each other again. You should aim to touch and caress each other with your hands in a way that is enjoyable for each other. If you are touching your partner, you should try to touch parts of the body that you have not explored before. I usually recommend that the genital areas and breasts remain "out of bounds" at this stage. This means that there is less chance of performance anxiety or of being worried about what will happen, because you both know that your intimacy will be restricted to sensual touching and caressing.

While you are being touched and caressed by your partner, try to concentrate on the sensations; relax and enjoy yourself, safe in the knowledge that enjoyable touching is all that will happen. Try to praise your partner when they do things that you like. You can do this in whatever way you wish—for example, by moving your partner's hand back for more of the caressing and touching you find most enjoyable. You can even demonstrate to your partner how you would like them to caress and touch you, and then lie back, relax, and enjoy it. If you don't like your partner touching a certain part of your body, then gently move their hand elsewhere. You may notice that these touching sessions make you aroused. If you feel comfortable with the idea, you could masturbate as a response to the arousal. I usually advise couples not to move on from the gentle caressing and touching stage until they are both comfortable and relaxed during such intimate moments.

As you begin to feel less anxious about these moments of intimacy, the genitals and breasts need no longer be out of bounds. You can incorporate these areas of each partner's body into the caressing and touching. Remember that you should continue to give your partner feedback by guiding their hands and saying what is really pleasurable for you. In this stage of the graded intimacy program, which includes body parts like the penis and breasts, it is important that you not forget to include the other body parts. Some couples decide to add the use of body lotions and massage oils at this stage, to enhance the feelings of pleasure and intimacy. You may find that at this stage one of you becomes very aroused and may even experience an orgasm.

When you notice that the male in the partnership is getting a fairly hard erection, the woman may invite her partner to insert his penis into her vagina. The aim of this stage is to get used to the body sensation of the penis in the vagina (this is called vaginal containment). The best position for this is with the man lying on his back and the woman kneeling above him with her knees at either side of his nipples. Try to keep the penis in the vagina for about fifteen seconds—you can increase the time on each successive occasion if either of you is worried about going further. You should both try to concentrate on the sensations involved at this stage. Remember that the aim is to get used to each stage and to be comfortable before moving on to the next stage.

By the time you are ready to begin this final stage, you should each be touching each other in ways you both enjoy, with no particular performance in mind other than enjoying yourself and giving your partner a pleasurable, intimate experience. Different couples go through this graded program at different speeds. The speed doesn't matter as long as you move from one stage to the next only when you both feel comfortable. When this graded program is completed, you should feel ready to integrate sexual intercourse with the other components that you have worked through.

Pregnancy and Contraception

Many men with an ostomy have become fathers after ostomy surgery. Similarly, having an ostomy need not be an obstacle to a woman's becoming pregnant. Many, many women with ostomies have given birth to healthy babies. You may be advised to wait for a time after the ostomy operation before becoming pregnant. There are various reasons for this advice. It may be to enable you to get used to looking after the ostomy or so that your abdominal muscles get a chance to strengthen.

Oral contraceptive medication may not be fully effective when you have certain types of ostomies, especially an ileostomy. This is because the medication may not be absorbed as it should be. In these cases, you should ensure that you use other methods of contraception, such as condoms, to ensure maximum effectiveness. If you have any concerns or questions about contraception or family planning, contact your ET or doctor for further advice.

Summary

Ostomy patients are not always given information on sex and intimacy. Even though it can be challenging to overcome the embarrassment most of us feel at times about discussing these issues, talk to your doctor or nurse if you have concerns; she or he can offer suggestions, and you will soon feel more at ease.

If you are not in an intimate relationship when you have ostomy surgery, it can be difficult to know if, when, and how to tell a potential new partner that you have an ostomy.

If you are worried about telling someone you have an ostomy, it may be helpful to think through all your options in advance. When you have chosen an option, think about how you would deal with the other person's possible responses. If you do this, you will be prepared and won't need to worry about the unexpected; you will have thought of it already. Most people find that potential partners react well to being told about the ostomy.

If you are already in a relationship, you might be worried about how your relationship will be affected. The key to dealing with this is for you and your partner to talk to one another about how you both feel about life with an ostomy.

The human sexual response can be divided into five stages—desire, excitement, plateau, orgasm, and resolution. Problems can develop at one or more of these stages and may be due to physical or psychological factors, or a combination of the two.

After the ostomy operation, allow yourself to take things easy; reintroduce sex and intimacy into your relationship gradually.

Simple techniques can be used for some of the common sexual problems after ostomy surgery; these include trying different sexual positions or using a lubricant. Persistent problems can be helped by a health professional trained in psychosexual disorders.

Many couples have conceived after ostomy surgery. Having an ostomy need not be a barrier to having children.

Chapter 9

Back to Life

I live a full and normal life. I eat and drink what I want, I travel,
work full-time, have relationships with men, and try to live life
to the fullest.

Female ileostomy patient, age 25

A s you become more familiar with the ostomy-care appliance, begin to regain your strength, and understand your
emotional reactions and how your thoughts about the
ostomy might be influencing them, you will probably begin to fully
enjoy some of the activities that contributed to your enjoyment of
life before your ostomy—activities such as eating, sleeping, travelling, working, and playing sports. This chapter highlights some of
the issues regarding various aspects of your quality of life in general
and provides advice on how to prevent and overcome any problems or worries that may arise in these areas.

Diet

There is usually no need for a special diet following ostomy
surgery—unless your doctor has told you to follow a diet because
of a problem such as diabetes or high blood pressure. In general,

you are advised to stick to three meals a day. However, you may find that certain foods cause you problems, such as blockage or constipation, gas, odor, diarrhea, or a change in the color of the waste material. The most commonly given advice regarding eating and ostomy care is to avoid certain foods if they keep causing the same problem. Remember, though, that it may be a particular *brand* of food that is causing you the problem—as opposed to a particular *type* of food.

On pages 116 to 118 there are lists of foods that are commonly linked to various problems; referring to these lists may help you find the culprit. Also, remember that everyone is different and that some of these foods may cause you no problems at all. In the early weeks after your operation, you may have a problem with a particular food, but this may be a one-time occurrence that settles down as time goes on and as you get used to having an ostomy.

If you are having a problem and you suspect that it may be due to a particular food, I suggest that you experiment on three occasions to see what happens after eating it; record your results in the Food-Problem Diary (use the blank form on page 115). These experiments will show whether the problem is caused by a particular food or not. This means that you don't exclude something from your diet when it may not be the cause of the problem.

You need to make sure that you take a few days off between each of your food experiments. If you get the same reaction (e.g., gas or constipation) on each occasion after eating that particular type of food, your experiment suggests that this food is causing your particular problem.

Certain foods seem more likely to cause common problems. There are no guarantees of the kind of reaction any one individual will get; however, the next sections list some of the common culprits. If you are especially worried about your diet, you may wish to introduce these foods into your diet gradually to see how you get along with them.

Food-Problem Diary

Type of food:
  Problem to be investigated:

. . . .

  Experiment No. 1   Date: _____
  Result:

. . . .
. . . .

  Experiment No. 2   Date: _____
  Result:

. . . .
. . . .

  Experiment No. 3   Date: _____
  Result:

. . . .
. . . .

Have you noticed any pattern in your reaction to this food on each experiment?

. . . .
. . . .

After three experiments, what is your conclusion about this particular food? Remember to think about whether there are other factors that might have influenced this reaction.

. . . .
. . . .

Does this food seem to be the main cause of this particular problem?
  Yes / No

What action will you take now as a result of these experiments (e.g., exclude this food from your diet, do some more experiments to confirm the cause, speak to your ET, etc.)?

. . . .
. . . .

Make copies of this format for additional records

Gas

Various foods can contribute to causing gas (the technical term is flatus)—and some of us are born with a tendency to be more troubled with gas than others. Gulping food, talking while eating, smoking, skipping meals, and drinking soft drinks can also increase the chances of experiencing problems with gas. Certain foods and drinks also increase the chances for gassiness. These include

* alcohol

* beans

* broccoli

* brussels sprouts

* cabbage

* cauliflower

* chewing gum

* cucumber

* soft drinks

* milk

* mushrooms

* nuts

* peas

* spinach

* corn

* turnips

If you suffer from gas following the ostomy operation, there are a number of things you can do to minimize the problem. First, do your own experiments with different foods, and avoid any which are a problem. Make sure you chew your food well, keeping your mouth closed and waiting until you have swallowed one mouthful before you take another. It has been suggested that drinking fennel tea, eating two pineapple capsules (available in health food shops), eating a very ripe banana, or eating ten to twenty marshmallows can all be effective in helping with gas.

Change in Color

Sometimes you may notice that the waste material in the ostomy-care appliance has changed in color. This can be alarming if you don't realize that such changes can result from eating certain food-stuffs. The following foods are particularly likely to cause a change in the color of the waste that is collected by the ostomy appliance:

* beets

* blueberries

* iron pills

* licorice

* red food dye

* strawberries

If you notice a change in waste color, think back to see if you have eaten any of the foods listed above.

Odor

Some foods are associated with the production of smell and odor. If you have been bothered by an increase in the smell of your waste material, one of the following foods may be to blame:

* asparagus

* baked beans

* broccoli

* Brussels sprouts

* cabbage

* cauliflower

* cod liver oil

* cucumber

* eggs

* fish

* garlic

* onions

* peanut butter

* some spices

* strong cheese

If you are troubled by smells from a urostomy, you can put three drops (approximately one milliliter) of vinegar into the pouch to combat the odor. You should drink plenty of fluids when you have a urostomy and try to eat foods that are high in vitamin C; this reduces the chances of your getting a urinary tract infection and may also reduce the likelihood of smelly urine.

It has been suggested that certain foods can actually reduce odor; some people claim this is true of peppermint oil, yogurt, and buttermilk. A soluble aspirin or some vanilla essence can be placed in a colostomy or ileostomy appliance to help prevent troublesome odors.

Diarrhea

Diarrhea can be caused by highly spiced foods, beans, peas, prunes, raw fruit, chocolate, and spinach. It can also be caused by an increased consumption of alcohol and can sometimes result from increased mental and physical tension. If you have an ileostomy, you should be particularly aware of the foods that have been listed as causing diarrhea. It is also important to make sure that you drink large amounts of water and that you have plenty of salt in your diet.

It is a good idea to tell any doctor who is giving you medication that you have an ostomy. This is because the changes in your body's functioning may mean that drugs are absorbed in different ways—this is especially important if you are being troubled by diarrhea.

Blockage and Constipation

The warning sign of a blockage is when waste material is not produced for a longer interval than is usual for you. Sometimes the production of a watery fluid, and nothing else, is a signal that you have a blockage. As with any ostomy problems that you notice or are concerned with, you should contact your doctor or ET for advice. If you get a blockage, don't worry too much; blockages are usually sorted out easily with the proper medical attention. Celery, nuts, corn, and coconut are particular foods that may result in a blockage. You may need to avoid these if they keep causing you to have blockage problems.

Sleep

Sometimes people who have had an ostomy operation find that they have difficulties sleeping when they return home from the hospital. This can be due to the change in environment from the hospital and may be part of getting used to your own nighttime routine and bed again. It may also be due to worries that the ostomy appliance will leak during the night. Sleep problems can be major obstacles to your return to a happy and fulfilled life after ostomy surgery. Sleep has an extremely important function in restoring our energy and helping our bodies to recuperate. Getting a good night's sleep is therefore especially important following ostomy surgery, when your body and mind are recovering from a major operation. If you have difficulty sleeping and you want to establish a good sleep pattern, there are a number of rules you can follow to promote a good night's sleep.

Try to avoid heavy snacks before bedtime, and if you must have a drink, it is better to choose a hot, milky drink. Alcohol and caffeinated drinks—such as coffee, colas, and tea—should also be avoided before bedtime. These drinks increase arousal and can disrupt your sleeping pattern.

It may sound very basic to advise you that your bed and mattress should be comfortable and that the room temperature should be around 65° F. However, bed comfort and room temperature are important in promoting a healthy sleep pattern.

Try to remember that beds are for sleeping; they are not designed for watching TV, reading, or knitting. If we do these things in bed, our beds become linked in our minds with these activities rather than with sleeping. In other words, we start to develop the link "bed = TV = arousal," instead of "bed = rest = sleep." This means we find it more difficult to get to sleep, because we get used to being in bed when our minds and bodies are active. Here are some ways of getting around the problem of an overactive mind or body preventing sleep:

* Go to bed only when you are "sleepy tired."

* Try to wind down toward the end of an evening. You might want to set a deadline of refraining from "arousing" activity (physical or mental) for about an hour before going to bed.

* Some people cannot get to sleep because thoughts keep going around and around in their heads—thoughts about what they have been doing, what they will do the following day, worries about family, health, bills, etc. It often helps to write all these thoughts down on a piece of paper before you go to bed—then tell yourself that they are all there for you to pick up in the morning. There is nothing you can do about them overnight. I

sometimes use this strategy after a difficult day at work. I write down all the things that have to be done, the worries and the particular issues that need attention. Then I put the piece of paper in a drawer in my study, and I tell myself that I'll collect it in the morning before I go to work.

* When you get into bed, turn the light out immediately; do not read, watch TV, or engage in any other "waking" activity.

* Avoid trying too hard to fall asleep. You could say to yourself, "Sleep will come when it is ready" or repeat a calming phrase over and over in your mind, such as "I am rested, relaxed, and calm." If you are still awake twenty minutes later, get up and go sit and relax in another room. Remember that you are trying to associate bed with sleep, not tossing and turning, reading, or worrying. When you feel "sleepy tired" again, go back to bed (wait until you do feel this even if it takes a long time—you will get into a pattern eventually). If you do not get to sleep after another twenty minutes, keep repeating this routine until you establish a regular sleep pattern. You will develop a sleep pattern if you stick to this program.

* Set your alarm to go off at the same time every day.

* Make a rule not to take naps during the day and not to sleep during the day to "catch up" on lost sleep.

All of these elements are essential to developing a healthy sleep pattern.

Travelling with an Ostomy

There is no reason why you cannot travel at home or abroad when you have an ostomy. However, there are certain factors you would be wise to take into account before you travel. If you are flying, it is a good idea to take at least some of your ostomy-care appliances and equipment in your carry-on bag in case your checked luggage gets lost. Removing appliances from their boxes may give you more room in your suitcase (though be careful not to damage them). It is also generally recommended that you estimate how much ostomy-care equipment you will need—and then take twice this quantity with you. Taking more than you need means that you'll have enough supplies to cope with more frequent changing, delays to your journey, or problems with appliances that get damaged during the course of travel.

Travel-insurance policies often exclude preexisting medical conditions—and that includes matters relating to an ostomy. If you have a specific query relating to travel insurance, contact your ET or one of the ostomy-patient organizations, or ask your travel agent. You may be required to provide evidence of your ostomy in the form of a letter from your doctor

Customs officers know what ostomy appliances are. Hardly any ostomy patients are ever stopped, and those who have been stopped tell me they have had no problems. If you are travelling abroad, you will probably find it helpful to obtain a travel certificate (consult your health-care provider or one of the ostomy-patient organizations). These certificates outline in different languages what an ostomy involves and the steps that need to be taken to ensure that problems with missing luggage and body searches are minimized. Travel certificates usually contain information as follows:

To whom it may concern:

This is to certify that the person named on this certificate has had a surgical operation that makes it necessary for him/her to wear at all times a bag attached to the abdomen to collect excretion from the bowel or bladder. If it is necessary to examine this bag, a qualified medical practitioner should be present, because any interference may cause leakage and great discomfort and embarrassment to the wearer. The bag may be supported by a belt; if so, this may have metal parts that register on a metal detector. The owner of this certificate may also be carrying an emergency supply pack consisting of spare bags, surgical dressings, etc., in addition to his/her main luggage. It is essential that these emergency supplies remain intact and are not mislaid.

Travel certificates usually include translations of the message into several languages. If you need an explanation in a language not included on the certificate, contact an ostomy-patient association (see "Resources") or your doctor's office. They will help you obtain the information you need. Someone at your doctor's office can also give you details of how to contact an ET wherever you are travelling, at home or abroad.

Anyone travelling abroad, ostomate or otherwise, needs to take sensible precautions against what we in the UK call "holiday tummy." This is especially important if you have a colostomy or ileostomy. You should make sure that you carry antidiarrheal medication with you and that you drink only bottled water when on holiday abroad. If you have an ileostomy and are travelling to a hot country, you should be especially careful to avoid becoming dehydrated.

You may have concerns about staying overnight in places that are new to you. Your worries are likely to be focused on whether you have an accident and how you will deal with this. The worst-case scenario technique, described in Chapter 7, can help with these travel worries. If you are worried about leaks on bedclothes, take a special protective sheet with you. If you are worried about needing to change quickly in a strange environment, you could try to obtain a card explaining why you might need to use a toilet in a hurry. Your ET or an ostomy-patient organization (see "Resources") will be able to advise you on this.

Sports

You may be concerned that engaging in intense physical activity—including certain sports—could damage the ostomy. It is very difficult to injure an ostomy; ostomies are very resilient and resistant to damage. In addition to this general concern, some sports are associated with particular worries for ostomy patients. Swimming, for example, is a particularly good form of exercise but can pose specific problems to someone with an ostomy: worries that other people may notice the ostomy through the swimsuit, concerns that the appliance may fall off, or embarrassment about changing clothes in front of other people. Earlier chapters present suggestions that can help you deal with these concerns (such as Chapter 5, on modifying problem thoughts that other people may be able to detect the ostomy and the appliance).

When your ostomy appliance is exposed to water, the adhesive seal becomes even more secure, because the adhesive properties are enhanced by water. If you don't believe this, notice that your ostomy appliance is more difficult to remove in a bath. If this knowledge doesn't help, remind yourself when you have this worry that your appliance is being held in place by your swimsuit anyway. If, after challenging your thoughts that people can see your ostomy appliance through your swimsuit, you are still worried about this, then try wearing your swimsuit in the bathtub and have a look for yourself. How many people are going to be interested in what you are wearing? Do you look at the color, shape, and style of other people's swimsuits when you are at the pool? If not, then how likely is it that other people are watching you? Next time you are at the swimming pool, try to spot all the people with ostomies. This will help you see how difficult it is. You can also buy a patterned swimsuit and use a smaller appliance while you are swimming, if this would help you feel more comfortable and less concerned that other people will notice the appliance. Some swimming pools have restricted times for adults or quiet times; you might feel more comfortable going at those times until your confidence returns.

There are no easy answers to worries about changing clothes in front of other people. But there are some helpful strategies that can make it easier. You could get changed in a cubicle or dressing room or wear a long shirt over your suit. Some people cope with this worry by taking a sweatsuit, or something similar, to change into. They change into it when they leave the pool and then change out of their swimsuit when they get home.

If you are involved in other sporting activities, such as soccer or tennis, you should encounter no major problems once your ostomy is in place. You'll need to build up your fitness (just like anyone else after major surgery), and you can experiment with different solutions for keeping the appliance in place, such as wearing a special belt. If there is a risk of your ostomy being hit in contact sports, you should ask your ET about obtaining an ostomy guard.

Dehydration following physical activity can be a particular problem for people with an ileostomy or a urostomy. If you are involved in sports activities, it is important to make sure that you adequately replace any fluids lost.

Driving

Your ET or doctor will advise you as to when it is safe for you to drive after the ostomy operation. This is usually three or four weeks after surgery. It is not advisable to drive before then, as the physical activity involved (for example, in turning the steering wheel) may cause a problem with the ostomy. If you are worried about the position of the seat belt in relation to your ostomy, you can get a special device that keeps the belt off this area but still enables you to wear the belt safely. Such a device can be obtained from most automobile-accessory stores.

Work

With many of the general lifestyle issues following ostomy surgery, the advice is to take things easy and work gradually toward getting back to your old lifestyle. This means that you are working slowly and steadily toward a final goal, taking small steps to boost your confidence along the way. A helpful hint for worrisome, difficult, or new situations is to approach them in small steps (as described in Chapter 7). Any task is easier if it is broken down into smaller, manageable chunks than if you try to deal with it all at once. Once you have conquered one part of the task, you get a sense of achievement that will not only make you feel good but also spur you on to deal with the next step in the process. If you try to go for your ultimate goal right away, you increase the risk of being disappointed and giving up on it. You might also be less likely to try again in the future. This is an important process to remember as you plan your return to work after the ostomy operation.

Returning to work can be an important part of life with an ostomy—a major step in getting back to normal. Work provides structure to your day and gives you the opportunity to test how you are adjusting to life with your ostomy. You have to deal with changing the appliance, talking to other people, and doing all the things you would usually do at work. Make sure you don't go back to work too early, as this may cause further problems. You may lack enough energy to go back full-time right away, or you may be worried about how you will manage. Going back part-time to start with can be very helpful for testing your stamina and coping with any worries you may have.

Some jobs might be unsuitable for someone after an ostomy operation (for example, jobs involving heavy lifting). It is usually possible for an employee to discuss with his or her employer any problems resulting from the surgery and to come to an agreement allowing the employee to work without risking injury. Your doctor or nurse can advise you on any aspects of your work situation that might need to be discussed with your employer. These professionals can also contact your employer if you think their doing so might help you.

Summary

You shouldn't experience major troubles with diet after ostomy surgery. But certain foods can cause problems such as diarrhea, gas, and odor. Keep a note of when these problems happen, so that you can limit your intake of troublesome foods and thereby gain control over the problem.

Sleep is important in promoting physical and mental recovery from an ostomy operation. If your sleep pattern is disrupted, strategies exist to help you return your body to a proper sleep pattern. These include going to bed only when you are "sleepy tired," avoiding reading or watching TV in bed, and dealing with worries before you get into bed.

Travel with an ostomy means being prepared; this usually involves packing appliances, finding out the name of an ET in case of emergencies, and getting proper insurance and a travel certificate if you are travelling abroad.

There are no reasons why people with an ostomy cannot take part in sports—the ostomy does not get damaged, and most concerns you might have about sports, such as swimming, can be dealt with using practical coping strategies.

Returning to work following ostomy surgery can be difficult; it is therefore best to avoid going back too early. It is often better to try a gradual approach and to speak to your employer about your specific situation.

Afterword

This book was written to provide you with information that can help you to understand your experiences and correct any misconceptions that you may have about living with your ostomy. Extensive information has also been included about how to make optimal psychological adjustments after this form of major surgery, a dimension of ostomy care that is often overlooked.

Research suggests that positive adjustment to ostomy surgery is more likely to occur when you feel confident and in control. Identifying and challenging negative thoughts can alleviate the distress that is associated with negative thinking, anxiety, and depression. The information in this book should allow you to develop individual ways of dealing with the issues and feelings that come up and to make decisions based on a sound knowledge of the options available to you. In summary, tackling the challenges that you face in a step-by-step manner can greatly enhance your quality of life.

I hope that reading this book has helped you discover the many positive options that exist for you as you live your life with an ostomy.

Resources

Charter of Ostomates' Rights

The Charter of Ostomates' Rights was issued by the International Ostomy Association's Coordination Committee in June 1993 (rev. June 1997). It is printed here for your information. Since this is not a U.S. organization, the word "stoma" is used in place of "ostomy."

It is the declared objective of the International Ostomy Association that all ostomates shall have the right to a satisfactory quality of life after their surgery and that this charter shall be realized in all countries of the world.

Ostomates shall:

* Receive preoperative counselling to ensure that they are fully aware of the risks and benefits of the operation and the essential facts about living with a stoma.

* Have a well-constructed stoma placed at an appropriate site, and with full and proper consideration to the comfort of the patient.

* Receive experienced and professional medical support and stoma nursing care in the preoperative and postoperative periods both in hospital and in their community.

* Receive full and impartial information about all relevant supplies and products available in their country.

* Have the opportunity to choose from the available variety of ostomy management products without prejudice or constraint.

* Be given information about their National Ostomy Association and the services and support which can be provided.

* Receive support and information for the benefit of family, personal careers, and friends to increase their understanding of the conditions and adjustments which are necessary for achieving a satisfactory standard of life with a stoma.

* Receive assurance that personal information regarding ostomy surgery will be treated with discretion and confidentiality to maintain privacy.

Useful Information

Ostomy-Patient Organizations

These organizations often have local contacts who can provide you with information on what they do and what support they might be able to provide before and after surgery.

International Ostomy Association (IOA)
c/o British Colostomy Association
15 Station Rd., Reading, Berkshire RG1 1LG , UK
Helpline: 011-44-1734-391537
Website: www.ostomyinternational.org

United Ostomy Association (UOA)
19772 MacArthur Blvd., Ste. 200
Irvine CA 92612-2405
(800) 826-0826   (949) 660-8624
Fax: (949) 660-9262   E-mail: director@uoa.org
Website: www.uoa.org

Appliance Manufacturers

These are the names and addresses of some of the main appliance manufacturers in the United States. Most of them have toll-free telephone numbers with trained staff to advise on appliances and ostomy care.

Coloplast, Inc.
5610 W. Sligh Ave., Ste. 100-C
Tampa FL 33634   (800) 237-4555

ConvaTec, Inc.
PO Box 5254
Princeton NJ 08543   (800) 422-8811

Cymed Ostomy Co.
1336 A Channing Way
Berkeley CA 94702   (800) 582-0707

Dansac Products (by Incutech, Inc.)
PO Box 1608
Kernersville NC 27285   (800) 699-4232
Website: http://store.yahoo.com/incutech/index.html

Hollister, Inc.
2000 Hollister Dr.
Libertyville IL 60048   (800) 323-4060

Torbot Ostomy and Medical Supply
Torbot Group, Inc.
1367 Elmwood Ave.
PO Box 3564
Cranston RI 07910   (800) 545-4254

Other Useful Contacts

King Medical Supply
431 W. 13th Ave.
Eugene OR 97401   (800) 207-8322
(541) 345-0391   Fax: (541) 345-0392
Website: www.kingmedical.qpg.com
A home-health-care supply company specializing in ostomy supplies. It offers specialty products including Whoo-Noz deodorant tablets (ileostomy), Odor-Cide liquid deodorant (urostomy), and customized nonadhesive systems.

Nu-Hope Laboratories, Inc.
12640 Branford St.
Pacoima CA 91331   (800) 899-5017
Produces customized ostomy supplies, including ostomy support belts and custom precut openings.

Wound, Ostomy and Continence Nurses Society (WOCN)
1550 S. Coast Hwy., Ste. 201
Laguna Beach CA 92651   (888) 224-9626
Fax: (949) 376-3456   Website: www.wocn.org
A professional, international society for nurses specializing in the care of wound, ostomy, and continence patients. Contact this organization for information and local referrals of ostomy nurse specialists.

American Cancer Society (ACS)
(800) ACS-2345 (227-2345)   Website: www.cancer.org
A nationwide organization dedicated to eliminating cancer as a major health problem and diminishing suffering from cancer. A variety of ser-

vice and rehabilitation programs are available to cancer patients and their families. Contact ACS for your local chapter; chapters exist all over the country.

Resources for Health-Care Professionals

Health-care professionals who are interested in obtaining copies of materials used in this book (e.g., Appliance Confidence Monitoring Form, Appliance Trials Monitoring Form, Food-Problem Diary, etc.) to promote adjustment to ostomy surgery should contact

> Dr. C. A. White
> Department of Psychological Medicine, University of Glasgow
> Academic Centre, Gartnavel Royal Hospital
> 1055 Great Western Rd.
> Glasgow, G12 0XH, Scotland, UK.

Further Reading

Greenberger, D., and C. A. Padesky. *Mind over Mood: Changing How You Feel by Changing the Way You Think*. New York: The Guilford Press, 1996.

Mullen, B. D., and K. A. McGinn. *The Ostomy Book: Living Comfortably with Colostomies, Ileostomies and Urostomies*. Boulder, CO: Bull Publishing, 1992.

Northover, J. M. A., and J. D. Kettner. *Bowel Cancer: The Facts*. Oxford, UK: Oxford University Press, 1992.

Ostomy Quarterly, a magazine published by the United Ostomy Association; subscription is included in annual membership dues, or can be purchased separately for $25.00 per year. For contact information see UOA under "Ostomy-Patient Organizations," above.

Index